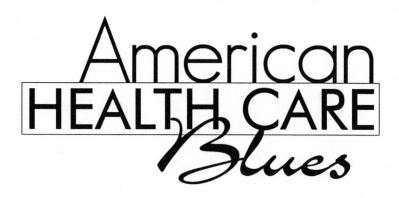

IRWIN MILLER

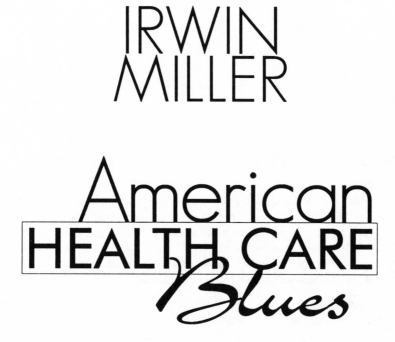

American HEALTH CARE Blues

Blue Cross,
HMOs, and Pragmatic
Reform Since
1960

TRANSACTION PUBLISHERS
New Brunswick (U.S.A.) and London (U.K.)

Library of Congress Catalog Number: 96-17334
ISBN: 1-56000-265-4
Printed in the United States of America

Library of Congress Cataloging-in-Publication Data

Miller, Irwin.
American health care blues : Blue Cross, HMOs, and pragmatic reform since 1960 / Irwin Miller.
p. cm.
Includes bibliographical references and index.
ISBN 1-56000-265-4 (alk. paper)
1. Blue Cross Association—History. 2. Insurance, Health—United States. 3. Insurance, Hospitalization—United States. 4. Health maintenance organizations—United States. 5. Medical policy—United States. I. Title.
HG9396.M55 1996
368.3'82'00973—dc20   96-17334
                                                                     CIP

*We thus abandoned, to a varying degree among the Plans,
the original philosophy and the basic concept of Blue Cross
as a community service organization... and took on the
trappings of commercial insurance.... But that need not
be our function or our destiny.... The task...is to restore
and put new life into an original concept.... We must
agree as to what we are and where we are going. We must
recapture the evangelistic spirit which characterized Blue
Cross in its youth. We in Blue Cross must steer our course
by the fixed stars of community service rather than by the
moving lights from the near-by shore of expediency or by
the contrary currents of commercial competition.*

—James Stuart
(Cincinnati Blue Cross CEO)
"Blue Cross Slips Are Showing"
(1953)

*Accordingly, I shall... inquire first what is the meaning in
general of a critical change in life.... Reconstruction [of
critical situations]... represents, in history, a conflict
between ideas and the institutions which embody those
ideas.... The [leader], the one who is for progress, cannot
gain his end if he shuts himself off from the established facts
of life. If he turns to the future before he has taken home to
himself the meaning of the past, his efforts will be futile....
The only force, the only instruments with which he may
carry out his projects of progress are the traditions, the
institutions of the past in their readjustment and reconstruction....The only final conservative force in life is
the most radical idea absorbed into the character which
has thus learned the lesson of the past. The most progressive force in life is the idea of the past set free from its
local and partial bonds and moving on to the fuller
expression of its destiny.*

—John Dewey
"Reconstruction" (1894)

Contents

1

Introduction:
Taking Home the Meaning of the Past

The Blue Cross and Blue Shield Association recently (October, 1993) came out with a little white policy paper called "A Pragmatic Approach to Health Care Reform." But what is a pragmatic approach to health policy and reform? A follow-up article by an Association executive provides as essential clue: pragmatic reform focuses on institution building (Cohodes, 1994). This book, using a Selznickian (and Deweyan) perspective, interprets Blue Cross diversification into HMOs as an exemplification of a pragmatic institution building approach to health policy and reform. A pragmatic (Deweyan) perspective is designed to deal with critical times and decisions that face society. It focuses on institutions and traditions as key tools for reconstruction. Leaders work such reform by mediating between past and future, between means and ends. They strive to give organizations moral character and they strive to build community.

This book tells the story of how the national trade association leaders of America's loose confederation of independent Blue Cross plans, the world's largest private health insurer, got their membership to diversify—in the face of local plan reluctance and national organized medicine resistance—into HMOs over a thirty-five year period (1960–1995). This radical shift (amidst the rapid erosion of the nonprofit ethos in our society in the 1980s) seemingly reconstructed the conservative Blues into a more viable enterprise both in the 1990s new managed care marketplace and unfolding national policy reforms. It also, however, dangerously eclipsed the Blues' guiding principle: "community service." Then in late 1990 a Blue Cross and Blue Shield Plan in West Virginia became insolvent. With this erosion came gnawing questions: Are the Blues self-destructing? Can they regain a worthy common mission and further seek

1

their community destiny? Can incremental change be progressive? Can leadership be responsible?

The book has five (perhaps six) main audiences. First, it is a case study of the role of leadership in the organizational development of one of America's largest service enterprises. Sociologists will be interested in this. Second, it is a case study of the recent 1960–1995 evolution of the world's largest private health insurer. Thus, it will hopefully be informative to those interested in what Blue Cross has been and its current identity crisis. (I especially hope Blue Cross and Blue Shield board members read it.) Third, this story of organizational adaptation sheds light on what a pragmatic (Deweyan) approach to health reform looks like. Thus, it may find a readership in both health policy and public policy circles. For to be a credible policy outlook pragmatism must mean something more than short-term practicality or the self-serving misdeeds of some Blue Cross plans unearthed by Senator Sam Nunn and his Sub-Committee on Investigations staff in recent years. Deweyan philosophy and sociology offer a constructive alternative meaning to a pragmatic approach to public policy, an approach that John Friedmann (1987) calls "the social learning" tradition. Fourth, as a rare longitudinal study of organizational leadership, it will be of interest to health care and other executives facing the challenges of institution building, renewal, and transformation. Fifth, as it offers a Deweyan interpretation of health care, it offers some facts and insights that communitarians may find of use.

A sixth possible audience are medical historians. Both Dewey and Selznick point in the direction of hermeneutics, that is, interpretive inquiry to better understand our presupposed way of understanding the world. This involves appreciating how traditions and rhetoric invest our institutions, policies, and efforts with meaning. As medical historian Daniel Fox (1993) argues, a better understanding of the past is essential to an adequate understanding of our present health policy situation and alternatives. And so, I have set the Blue Cross-HMO story in the historical context of a pragmatic tradition in health policy and reform, one founded by Benjamin Franklin when he served as the social architect of our first community hospital, Pennsylvania Hospital in Philadelphia. My aim, then, is to explore this pragmatic way of understanding and coping with social problems.

Recently, the Robert Wood Johnson Foundation (1995) has urged that health policy studies move beyond traditional single discipline, quantitative methods. This study is responsive to this call. It is qualitative and interdisciplinary. It focuses on the process of managing change and the role of leadership and rhetoric (ideological and utopian) in such change. It is anchored on Philip Selznick's institutional perspective, enlarging this approach by going back to Dewey's pragmatism and ahead to Paul Ricoeur's hermeneutics. This Selznickian study is like "an internal history" (Padgug, 1991), but one configured by a scholarly structure. While I am interested in what the national leaders "said, did and why" (Brown, 1991b), I am more interested in the meaningful consequences and future implications of their deeds and words. This is the focus of a future-oriented "hermeneutics of action" (Ricoeur, 1991). I have balanced the use of subjective oral histories and interviews with more objective sources such as corporate memos, reports, and other Blue Cross archival materials, as well as critical U.S. Senate Committee hearing reports. While my aim is not historiographical per se, perhaps medical historians will find something of use in my reconceptualization of the past in terms of a pragmatic paradigm.

One of the benefits of giving institution-focused policy studies a hermeneutical twist is that it will let us interpret the Blues both sympathetically and suspiciously. For we will critically evaluate Blue Cross in terms of its own pragmatic tradition and standard. Having said this, let me mark out some obvious limitations to this little book. It is not a complete history or sociology of Blue Cross. Like its two predecessors, this Blue Cross study is a focused case study. This one focuses on the role of leadership in policy-oriented institution building. The interested reader can gain a fuller appreciation of this unique American institution by consulting Odin Anderson's sympathetic *Blue Cross Since 1929* (1975), Sylvia Law's critical *Blue Cross: What Went Wrong?* (1974), and the 1991 issue of *The Journal of Health Politics, Policy and Law* that focuses on New York City's Blue Cross Plan.

This book focuses on how an organization's leaders guide its reconstruction, what Selznick (1983, 1992) calls "institution building"—adding moral value to the organization. Central to this creative process is the leaders' use of utopian language to redescribe problems in such a way as to persuade followers to enact novel solutions. In American health policy studies an emphasis on political rhetoric is doubly important, since for most of this century health reform has been debated in charged terms of political ideologies and utopias. Therefore to help clarify how pragmatic leaders use political rhetoric in health care institution building, I will offer a simple Deweyan set of six meanings of "policy," three being ideological (policy as ploy, pattern, and perspective) and three utopian (as plan, position and prod). My point here is that "policy" has five additional meanings beyond the assumed one of policy as a rational plan to achieve a goal.

This study explores questions such as:

*   What are the origins and reference points of a pragmatic American tradition of health care policy?;
*   How did the Blue Cross Association (BCA) come to endorse HMOs as public policy?;
*   What was the BCA approach to HMO public policy?;
*   What was the role of leadership and its rhetoric in this approach?;
*   How did the traditional Blue Cross confederation evolve into the nation's largest HMO system?;
*   What are the implications of this story for public policy for health care reconstruction in the future?;
*   What is Blue Cross' organizational character and destiny?

Dewey suggests that useful social criticism must rhetorically build outward from a society's tradition-funded identity. Therefore, after developing some elements of a pragmatic institution building approach to policy, I will provide in this chapter interpretations of three historical American reference points—instances of the exploration of the present's possibilities—to help guide our study of Blue Cross HMO policy: Benjamin Franklin's co-invention (1751) of the American community hospital, the Committee on the Costs of Medical Care (1927–32), and the emergence of Blue Cross (and prepaid group practice) (1929–1960). This historical interpretation will provide some insight into a pragmatic American health system and policy approach which I call policy as *prod*: the pragmatic exploration of the present's possibilities.

Chapter 2 will cover the 1960s, which prepared the way for the Blue Cross Association President Walter J. McNerney to propose a policy statement on prepaid group practice in 1970. In the 1960s McNerney exhorted about the radical prepaid group practice idea. Chapter 3 deals with the Blue Cross Association's, critical HMO policy decision which helped launch in the 1970s a movement of experimentation by some Blue Cross Plans to begin HMOs around the country. Chapter 4 covers the 1980s and 1990s, the consequence of McNerney's HMO strategy when the Blue

Cross HMO movement achieved significant marketplace success. Here the focus is on the consequences of the critical HMO decision on Blue Cross' organizational character. Chapter 5 looks to the future, offering a discussion of principles for reconstructing American health care.

This book began to percolate after my first book was published in 1984. In the late 1980s I decided to take my idea for a second book and incorporate it into my doctoral studies at The Union Institute. My dissertation committee was quite remarkable as it included Odin Anderson, Jack Salmon, and Frank Riessman, as well as Penny MacElveen-Hoehn, Barbara Perkins, and Fay McCutchan-Berglund. Their insights, criticisms and support were crucial to whatever strengths this book possesses. James Block's questions about chapter 1 helped me to better organize my argument. I would also like to thank the leadership of the Blue Cross and Blue Shield Association (where I worked on HMOs in the mid-1970s) for providing access to the organization's archives in 1990. I want also to thank present and past Association executives and other related officials for allowing me to interview them for this book (some of whom I worked with when I helped develop a Blue Cross approach to HMO building in the mid-1970s). Also, thanks go to Laurence Mintz for editing the book and to Linda Kuester for typing the manuscript. Finally, I dedicate this book to Ellen, Sophia, Nanny, and the Underfoots for their support during this book's evolution.

A Pragmatic Approach to Health Policy

This study looks at the Blue Cross Association's (BCA) voluntary, institution building approach to HMO policy as an example of what John Friedmann (1987) calls "the social learning tradition" of public policy studies. This tradition is based on John Dewey's pragmatic philosophy and Deweyan organization theory and sociology. Both focus on understanding action within particular situations. The pragmatic perspective is contingent, contextual and historical. *This tradition is pledged to the democratic exploration of the present's possibilities.* Social reconstruction— an experimental process—has five basic steps (Campbell, 1995). First, we detect that an aspect of our social set-up has ceased to work properly; doubt, conflict, anxiety are experienced. We have a felt need. Second, this felt need is recognized, taken up, as a problematic situation. The indeterminate feeling of step one is given some definition. It is interpreted as something that needs inquiry and resolution. This definition of the situation, if "well put" (Dewey quoted in Campbell, 1995, p. 48) gets the inquiry off in the right direction. Our *take* of the situation, our consideration of it from various viewpoints, is suggestive of where to look for solutions. It is crucial here to incorporate many perspectives on the situation, to listen to others. The third step is that of social inquiry in which the situation, its constituent elements and their transactions are all studied. This process leads to step four, a suggested social change—a working hypothesis—is put before the public. This action and its consequences are evaluated by the public as step four. Step five is the acceptance of workable changes. The problem has been solved and doubt, anxiety, and so on, are settled for the time being. Notice that problems and solutions will only be taken up for consideration and action if inquiries and publics are *taken* with them, that is, captivated by them. In part, this is a function of how well they are "put," that is, the degree to which the inquiry's rhetoric effectively projects its interpretation of the situation and its possibilities.

We need to note, for the purpose of our study here, that Dewey (and his colleague and fellow pragmatist, James H. Tufts) stressed the central role of institutions in any society—and the need to ameliorate social problems by reconstructing social institutions (Campbell, 1992). This emphasis on institution building was imported into the social learning approach in Perlmutter's (1965) monograph *Towards a Theory and Practice of Social Architecture: Building Indispensable Institutions* which relied heavily upon Selznick's (1983) *Leadership in Administration: A Sociological Interpretation* which was first published in 1957.

Selznick has suggested that "leadership as statesmanship" (1983, p. 37) happens as organizations are transformed "into institutions and into agencies of community" (1992, p. 231). He calls this process "institution building" (1992, p. 232). He casts "organizations" within a mechanical metaphor: they are expedient and expendable tools. An institution is—using an organic metaphor—"understood as a product of social adaptation." Institutions, by having an inspiring moral character win peoples' loyalty. To convert a characterless organization into a distinctive institution, the leader "infuses [it] with value" (1992, p. 233). This infusion of values involves using symbolic language and building coalitions. Institutions have moral character. Critical decisions are those that have decisive consequences for an institution's moral character and identity.

Selznick provides an example: "[T]he more concerned we are about the assimilation of banking to ordinary business, with a loss of distinctive commitments to "savers" (as distinguished from "customers" or "investors"), the more relevant will be a focus on institution building" (1992, p. 233). Institutions become agencies of community as they become a way of our living meaningfully together—a participatory mode of democratic association (1992, p. 243, 501–3). In times of critical change, statesmen help their organizations and communities find themselves, adapt and flourish by replacing what Selznick calls worn out "defensive ideologies" (1983, p. 15 and 18) with healthy utopian moral visions which Selznick calls "myths" (1983, p. 151–52). Leadership's myth-making, utopian rhetoric, then, lies at the core of what Selznick calls, "the art of institution building" (1983, p. 152). Institution building is a process over time, one that falls into incremental phases.

To get a handle on how pragmatic statesmen use ideological and utopian rhetoric in institution building, let me move back to Selznick's source, the philosophy of John Dewey. Unfortunately, although Dewey's philosophy points to a need for a social hermeneutics, he did not provide one (Kloppenberg, 1986; Ross, 1991). He does provide some essential clues for a pragmatic social hermeneutical template—a set of different views of "policy." (Developing a full-fledged social hermeneutical approach to social inquiry and policy is a task beyond this book's scope or needs.) These clues are in Dewey's ideas about ends, means, radicalism, conservatism, pragmatic social reconstruction, and its distortions.

Dewey's ideas about "ends" (e.g., aims, purposes, ideals, ideologies, utopias) provide a clue about the sort of theory of social interpretation that would be consistent with his thought. The key is that for Dewey ends are tools (i.e., means) of the imagination for use in the present; ends are not something fixed. He called ends as tools "ends-in-view." Ends-in-view, he argues "influence present deliberation and...finally bring it to rest by furnishing an adequate stimulus to overt action. Consequently, ends arise and function within action" (1964, p. 70). An end-in-view, then, is a prod to experimentation, deliberation, and action. Ideals open up the present's possibilities for exploration (Dewey, 1991). When U.S. Representative Marty Russo (Illinois), for example, introduced a national health insurance proposal in Congress his end-in-view was to, in his words, "*spur* debate...and move us closer to solving our health care crisis" (Locin, March 7, 1991, Sec. 3, p. 3, Italics added). He saw his policy proposal as a prod to stimulate innovative discussion and action.

Dewey was critical of fixed ends—"ends-in-themselves"—and past custom because they could be used to both manipulate situations to serve particular interests and to divert attention from the constructive exploration of actual situations and consequences. For him, "the task of intelligence is to grasp and realize genuine opportunity, possibility" (1964, p. 78). Further, he warned about separating means and ends. Useful ends must be realizable, hence they must be imagined in the context of practical means. When ends are offered without connection to means "there is a so-called 'ideal' which is utopian and a [mere] matter of fancy" (1964, p. 106). We need, then, a future-oriented social hermeneutics that sees something good in views of society that can be tools of construction, of exploring possibilities, while warning us about the dangers of views that hide possibilities, serve vested interests, or are flights of fancy.

"Conservatism" and "radicalism" are two basic ways of viewing society and policy in Dewey's social philosophy (Feffer, 1993). "Conservatism" is what we generally think of as ideology-driven. To stress means over ends is to be ideological; to stress ends and ignore means is to be utopian. As Feffer (1993) points out Dewey temporally distinguishes these two outlooks. Ideology is defensive and past-oriented; utopia is change-embracing and future-oriented. Pragmatism mediates the two in present on-going efforts of social reconstruction, that is, the experimental and democratic search for worthy ends and effective means. The hazard of utopianism is a foolish disregard for finding workable means to realize lofty ideals. The hazard of ideology is to stick with obsolete traditional forms when new times require new solutions. Further, Dewey pulls utopia and ideology into one framework. He writes: "The strength of each school is the weakness of its opponent" (in Feffer, p. 169). Ideology and utopia need each other. Dewey opposes several other outlooks or methods to his of social experimentation and reconstruction:" authority...caprice, ignorance, prejudice and passion" (1925, p. 353).

Paul Ricoeur's *Lectures on Ideology and Utopia* (1986) provides a social hermeneutics consistent with these Deweyan ideas about social reconstruction. Symbolic mediation and rhetoric are, for Ricoeur, fundamental to both language and social action. Since policy is language about social action, it is, I suggest, also fundamentally symbolic and rhetorical. Like Dewey, Ricoeur contrasts and mediates ideology and utopia: ideology defends the past while utopia projects into the future. Let me review Ricoeur's argument and combine it with Dewey's insights.

At the conceptual level, Ricoeur suggests, ideologies are distorted ideas or pictures of reality. Here ideas create what Dewey might call artificial *ignorance*. At the level of symbolic meaning ideology is more basically a representation of reality. Ideology here does the healthy work of helping integrate society by preserving its identity. Dewey's *prejudice* understood as prejudgments marks this level. Between these levels of concept and symbol is a middle level of power and *authority*. Here ideology's function is to provide legitimacy to the status quo, to established interest groups.

Ricoeur builds a parallel analysis of utopia—Dewey's radicalism. At the conceptual level its pathological function is madness, capricious escape, what Ricoeur calls "the magic of thought" (p. 296). Under the spell of utopia's magical ends we *capriciously* ignore the messy problem of how to get from the status quo to the imagined alternative future—we ignore Dewey's warning to connect ends with practical means. The field of action is magically friction-free. Obstacles become unreal. Goals do not conflict. Transition is unproblematic in the capricious world of radical flights of fancy. At the power level utopia challenges what ideology legitimates: the authority of the status quo. Dewey's call for social *passion* to be used to change society's status quo is an example of utopia as challenge. Key here is that there is a reversal of motivation. Utopia at the power level attempts to impassion society—to move it. Some creative mind is called upon to be an intellectual gadfly for social change. At the healthy symbolic level utopia is "the exploration of the possible" (Ricoeur, 1986, p. 310), what Dewey thought of as experimenting with the possibilities of the present. What ideology cloaks, utopia reveals: the contingency of social life. Things can be otherwise. Utopia's dream here becomes a practical tool: something to be used to begin to change reality.

Ricoeur, like Dewey, suggests that we use utopia's health to correct for ideology's pathology. Thus, utopia can unmask and challenge ossified ideology. Further, ideology can anchor utopia's dangerous flights of fancy. Moreover, preservation of identity and exploration of the possible can work productively together. Mixing healthy and political forms of ideology and utopia constructively combines ends and means.

These six attitudes have their counterparts in terms of "policy." Mintzberg (1987) suggests that there are five different uses of the term "policy" (or "strategy"). First, there is policy as *plan*. This is a rational set of steps that lead to reaching a clearly defined goal. Where plan is a master blueprint it is an expression of utopian magical thinking. Next comes *perspective* which is an established mindset or world view. This correlates with ideology's integrative function. Then there is *pattern*; policy is revealed in an established pattern of behavior. Here we are at the ideological level of justifying the established authorities and interests in society. Also there is policy as *ploy*. This is the Machiavellian world of deception. A plan for example, is deployed not to help get you from A to B, but to distract your opponent's attention while you move towards C. Here ideological concepts distort our perception of society. Finally, policy can be *positioning*. Here policy moves you about—repositions you—in a problematic environment out of harm's way or towards windows of opportunity. This correlates to realizable utopian challenges to the society's status quo. To these five uses I would add a sixth, policy as pragmatic *prod*: a tool to stir up discussion and experimental action. Here you might present a proposal not with the intention of reaching its goal, but with the hope of arousing productive debate, enlightenment, and exploratory action. This is a utopian exploration of the present's possibilities.

Now, let us review three historical reference points in the evolution of the pragmatic tradition of health care thinking and doing to see if we can in Dewey's (1894) words take home to ourselves the meaning of the past. The first of these points is Benjamin Franklin's ingenious invention of American health care voluntarism when he concocted Pennsylvania Hospital (in 1751) out of the materials he found at hand: community need, leadership and action, competition between city and hinterland, and potential partnership with government. Exploring Franklin's chameleon-like personality and experimental style of civic institution building will help us understand what Rosemary Stevens has described as the American community hospital's "chameleon-like" (1989, p. 360) versatility. Our guiding clue to understanding Franklin and his approach to institution building will be seeing him, as Ketchum (1966) has suggested, as Dewey's precursor. Franklin was the first practitioner of the social learning approach. Next I will examine the Committee on the Costs of Medical Care (CCMC, 1927–1932). Here we will sort out the rhetorical public policy battle to define the health care situation of that era—the various dimensions of ideology and utopia put into play. The CCMC with its pragmatic sociological concern with community surveys and local experimentation will be interpreted both as following in Franklin's footsteps and as an early twentieth century instance of the pragmatic social learning approach to public policy study. Third, I will provide a brief interpretation of the evolution of Blue Cross from 1929 to 1960, paying special attention to the role of pragmatic leadership in Blue Cross institution building during this period.

Benjamin Franklin

Benjamin Franklin is an essential American reference point for health policy considerations (see Miller, 1993). He co-founded the first of our unique American community not-for-profit hospitals. In doing this he anticipated the social learning public policy approach in his action-oriented stress on community institution building and constructive use of rhetoric in such civic enterprise. He was a venturesome practitioner of pragmatic science who applied this method to social and natural problems alike. Franklin's attitude to civic issues was "let the experiment be made" (Quoted in Ketchum, p. 199). He had a basic conviction that people have a talent for working social reform by means of institution building (Ketchum).

It is essential to understand Franklin's chameleon-like nature and leadership style since much of American health care falls under his shadow. His pragmatic character and actions generated the ambivalent versatility, noted by Rosemary Stevens (1989), of America's voluntary health care institutions. These versatile institutions combine and recombine the good and bad aspects of ideology and utopia. The methods for creating civic decision-making networks that were mobilized to form the physician-community coalitions necessary to build local hospitals in the 200 years that followed Franklin's founding of Pennsylvania Hospital (Starr, 1982) were first spelled out in Franklin's widely read *Autobiography* (Franklin, 1961). There he described how he catalyzed the formation of America's first community, not-for-profit hospital. The curious chameleon-like ability of the twentieth-century American hospital to reinvent itself to meet shifting social needs (Stevens, 1989) had its origins in Franklin's invention and immediate re-invention of Pennsylvania Hospital.

Franklin poses a challenge to his friends and critics alike because he was so loosely attached to utopian theories or ideological doctrines. Van Doren called him a "harmonious human multitude" (quoted in Wright, 1986, p. 11). For Balzac, he was "the inventor of the lightning rod, the hoax, and the Republic." Lacking George Washington's *gravitas* (Wright, p. 3), his contemporaries, it was said, did not allow him to write the Declaration of Independence lest his wit cause him to hide a joke somewhere in the document. He was in Selznick's terms a masterful role player. The French nobility and philosophers called him the "chameleon octogenaire" as he charmed them all as the Colonies' coonskin-capped trickster, New World sage, and diplomat (Wright, p. 349).

Franklin had, as a young man, a bumptious style of leadership and debate. He then switched to a posture of affable civility, what Breitwiser calls, Franklin's "strategic humility" (1984, p. 236). This helped him avoid adopting or appearing to adopt, extreme ideological or utopian positions. It also helped him shift the focus away from his role as catalyst, and towards the contributions of others. Thus, he hid his own power in order to empower others, that is, to prod them into action.

Franklin's chameleonlike detachment, however, led some people into suspecting that his seeming disinterest, on the one hand, masked self-interest and a secret agenda, while on the other hand threatened to lead them into some capricious folly. Thus, Franklin's style in some minds raised the twin pathological dangers of ideology and utopia (Wright). Meanwhile, he was valorized because his actions produced civic benefits. His liminality, his plasticity, was always ingeniously in the service of his community, first, Philadelphia, and later America (Ketchum, 1966). For Franklin, being an exemplary American statesperson, then, involved being adroit at using tools found in a problematic situation, including principles and doctrines (Wright, 1986). His levitas had loyalty as a compass. He wanted to be "a useful citizen" (Wright, p. 6).

Breitwiser (1984) shows how Franklin consciously made himself into a representative self, that is, the exemplary New World Man. This took the form of the critical and constructive Yankee who tackled the world, not with authority and prejudice, but with ingenuity and civility (Breitwiser, 1984; Wright, 1986). He did this to give his bumptious fellow Americans a workable sense of meaningful common identity (Breitwiser, 1984). He fashioned his actions with the goal of creating a representative life. He strove to become a symbol of America. Moreover, he was a man of social action, not theory. As Franklin said, "well done is better than well said" (quoted in Wright, 1986, p, 26).

What then did Franklin exemplify? He was voluntary association and pragmatic action man par excellence. He was an institution builder. Max Weber, however, in his early book, *The Protestant Ethic and the Spirit of Capitalism* (1958) used Franklin as the best example of calculative, self-centered capitalistic man. Weber criticized Franklin and America for lacking any higher moral purpose beyond functional economic gain and for fleeing into trivial voluntary associations rather than confronting capitalism's conflicts of everyday life and politics. This interpretation misses quite a bit. Late in his career, Weber in *The Sociology of Religion* (1964) made a powerful distinction between two kinds of prophetic leadership. First, was the exemplary prophet who preached no doctrine but who lived out a certain pattern of life that others used as a worthy example to imitate. Second, was the ethical prophet of principles who had an explicit doctrine. This leader issues a set of articulated ethical principles that others could adopt and obey. Weber, in this context, had interpreted Franklin as an ethical prophet of clear capitalistic principles. This missed Franklin's goal of becoming an exemplary prophet, a representative self, of voluntary social action. Franklin had intended his public life to be taken as an example, one which transcended any of his *Poor Richard* ethical maxims. This brings to mind Dewey's favoring of moral prophets over moral codes.

James Luther Adams (1986) provides an exemplary prophetic view of Franklin. He sees Franklin as exemplifying the substantive side of the Protestant ethic. Adams stresses the Protestant's general institution building vocation of criticizing established institutions and building new ones that better serve the community as a whole. Such activities bundle together into associational movements for social change that "represent the institutional gradualization of revolution" (Adams, 1986, p. 117). Voluntary associations that are truly community-minded offer a way out of bureaucracy's monolithic maze. Adam argues that the hallmark of democratic society is the freedom to form or belong to voluntary associations that can conduct social innovation or criticism. He defines voluntarism as a participatory institutional concept "in which the individual through association with others gets a piece of the action. In its actual articulation it involves an exercise of power through organization" (1986, p. 173). This process involves power struggles as part of reshaping institutions and the distribution of power. It operates at the level of policy as prod and position.

Participation, moreover, Adams argues, in such voluntary organizations, provides people with experiences that widen their social imagination and equips them with political skills such as listening, discussing, and organizing. Voluntarism is, in short, a school of democracy that provides the skills vital for the institutionalization of gradual revolution. Voluntary associations are, then, a dispersed mechanism of social change and control, of piece-by-piece transformation. Adams calls this "the meroscopic" approach which attacks strategic elements of a problematic situation (p. 134).

In many ways Franklin embodies Ricoeur's (1986) notion of the political educator who acts as a civic gadfly, leading his community on a expedition into the possible. Similarly, Franklin brings to mind Dewey's stress on the need for social criticism, where the critic is neither inside a society's culture, nor outside it, but as Alexander (1987) suggests (borrowing Edward Said's term) "close to" it. Dewey wrote about the adventure of exploring the possibilities that exist "at the growing edge of things" (Dewey, 1958, p. 144). Here an autobiographical story told by Franklin to a friend is emblematic. While on a ride during a visit with friends in Maryland, he spotted a "whirlwind" moving across the landscape. He recalls that "The rest of the company stood looking at it, but my curiosity being stronger, I followed it, riding *close by* its side" (Franklin, 1961, p. 226, italics added). Later, he rejoined the group, teasingly asking them if such little tornadoes were common in their part of the country. As an explorer of the possible, Franklin was able to distance himself from his culture—to be "close by" the flux of the unknown, and then return "close to" his culture—equipped with some critical comment. For Franklin, social action began with criticism of the established order's shortcomings.

Criticism for Franklin led to institution building. Wright (1986) observes, "Franklin reached democratic solutions not from any collectivist or utopian dogma, but from a pragmatic, self-help orientation" (p. 80). Usually he was not the inventor of new civic institutions, but rather played the role of community institution midwife and civic promoter. He had a disaffection for ideological causes; his talent was in concocting creative compromises. He believed that a citizenry stimulated and informed by a process of public discussion would participate in civic institution building. He had great faith in persuasively presented facts. Beyond that, he was willing to engage in power politics to maneuver new institutions into being. This political cunning made him more potent than many twentieth-century progressives would later become.

Franklin's experimental approach to civic amelioration started with finding someone with a civic discontent (Ketchum, 1966). Then he would network around this person or problem. This led to a democratic process of problem-solving. He was a natural rebel against the status quo, but as

Ketchum (1966) points out, Franklin lacked any ideological or utopian passion for the best solution or policy. He strove to accomplish the best workable solution under current conditions (Ketchum). His pragmatism, like Dewey's was situation-shaped. He avoided any rigid or fanciful search for perfection. For him, people were master tool users and makers, that is, they were not slaves to any one tool or profession. His dedication to community improvement was his touchstone. It pushed him beyond the ideological status quo, but well short of utopian fanciful perfection.

There is an American approach to philanthropy, Boorstin (1987) argues, that flows from Franklin's concept of community service. Benjamin Franklin is its patron saint because he combined "business sense with an eye on the community" (Boorstin, 1987, p. 204). Franklin reconstructed "charity." Charity for Franklin was a prudent social act. It was no longer the traditional idea to benefit the giver's soul, but now to solve a social problem. Philanthropy in his approach was circular. Community-driven philanthropy puts the recipient in a position to contribute to the enlargement of the community by equipping him to be a productive worker. It was a process of empowerment. Such enlightened self-interest impelled Franklin to lead civic projects that included starting Pennsylvania Hospital, the American Philosophical Society, the University of Pennsylvania and the local volunteer fire department. For Franklin, Boorstin notes, the public/private distinction hardly existed. Government program and voluntary action were both agencies of community. They were tools to be used for the common good.

Drucker provides a provocative illustration of this practical utopianism from how Japanese policymaking politics today works. He observes that while the Japanese have enough interest group selfishness "to make a Tammany boss blush" (1981, p. 86), leaders there have to begin their deliberations with questions about the public policy consequences of their corporate strategic proposals. He argues that if any private organization there "wants to be listened to and to have influence on the policy making process, it must start out its own deliberations by considering the national interest, not its own concerns" (p. 86). The general point is that private planning needs to fit itself into a larger, public framework. This, of course, is very close to Selznick's notion of leadership which he ties to seeing things in larger community frameworks.

After initially floating the new community hospital idea, Dr. Thomas Bond asked in 1750 for Franklin's help in creating America's first voluntary hospital which would be modeled somewhat after the new hospitals that had been recently started in England. (In this section I rely on Franklin's [1961] account and Williams [1976] history of Pennsylvania Hospital.) Franklin reviewed and endorsed Bond's plans. Moreover, he agreed to lead a community fund-raising drive. Given his strategic location in Philadelphia society, with contacts to the general public, the elite and the professions, Franklin was a catalytic power broker who could put together coalitions to build institutions. He triggered a bandwagon. He used his newspaper to "prepare the minds of people" (Franklin, 1961, p. 133) and his personal contacts to reach the rich and the professional class.

When publicity and networking did not raise enough voluntary contributions to build the hospital, Franklin relied on a political maneuver to prod both the public and then politicians into giving more money. He reinvented his proposed private hospital as a public-private partnership. Basically, people in Philadelphia were tied to a health care status quo and people in other parts of Pennsylvania could not see enough benefits for them in the proposed urban-based hospital. Franklin simply invented his way out of the impasse. He invented the matching grant. He suggested that the state legislature—reflecting the countryside—match private donations coming mostly from the city. If two thousand pounds were privately raised, then government would, he proposed, match that sum with public funds.

The constructive mediatory trickery was this: Franklin reasoned, correctly as it turned out, that the state representatives would take up his suggestion and thereby gain considerable political credit by appearing as generous, caring fellows—while being confident that Philadelphian inertia would prevent the local 2000 pounds from being raised. The representatives felt that there was little chance that they would have to pay for their apparent generous offer. They saw his proposal as a way to cloak their investment in the status quo. Meanwhile, Franklin judged, again correctly, that Philadelphians would be prodded into action by the promise of getting a pound from their country rivals for every pound they cooperatively raised in the city. He repositioned their self-interest into a public channel. This is how four thousand pounds were raised. Franklin was delighted by his deft trickery: "I do not remember any of my political maneuvers, the success of which gave me at the time more pleasure; or that in after-thinking of it, I more easily excused myself for having made use of cunning" (Franklin, 1961, p. 134).

Notice that in order to build this institution he undogmatically moved the proposed hospital from being a private, nonprofit institution to being largely private, but with public financing—that is, a hybrid. He had thereby reinvented the American community hospital even before it was built. A chameleonlike genius thereby created the chameleonlike voluntary hospital, an institution that by its origin and nature could be continually reinvented—repositioned along a public/private continuum—to get a changing community task done. As Boorstin notes about Franklin: "If an activity was required and was not yet performed by a government...he thought it perfectly reasonable that individuals club together to do the job, not only to fill the job, but also *prod* or shame governments into doing their part" (1987, p. 204, italics added).

The Committee on The Costs of Medical Care

The Committee on the Costs of Medical Care (CCMC) was a vast foundation-funded research project on the nation's health care situation. It was begun in the "roaring twenties" (1927) and issued its findings in the early years of the Depression (1932). Interestingly, although the 1920s were heyday Republican years of apparent plenty, workers had been hard hit by hospital costs in the 1920s (Stevens, 1989). The Committee was composed largely of academic physicians and representatives from organized medicine. It was staffed by social scientists. It operated in the Progressive style of full confidence in the expert, research, cooperation and fact-finding. This was Franklinian. It had a bewildering disregard for political feasibility and implementation planning. This was quite un-Franklinian. It was blind to the political dimension of ideological power (Anderson, 1985; Starr, 1982). Its majority report recommended that the nation shift to group practice, group hospital prepayment and regional health care planning. A minority issued a dissenting report reflecting the conservative AMA viewpoint (Anderson, 1985; Stevens, 1971).

The majority report's recommendations were complex in their rhetoric. It made its case in terms of a "rational" model of social change developed by one of its social scientists. It characterized the problem as originating in the "lag between scientific advance and popular application" (Committee on Cost, 1932, p. 2.). The metaphor was that of "cultural lag" (Fox, 1986). In this view, American health care was lagging behind the various European systems because American private practice physicians were resisting inevitable adjustment to scientific and technological forces. Physician competence was challenged. This polarized the issue by blaming the key power group, the American fee-for-service solo practitioner (Fox, 1986). Moreover, some of the Committee used the lag metaphor as a radical utopian viewpoint, rejecting incremental change short of total health care reorganization and national health insurance (Fox, 1986).

The AMA's scattered attacks on health care reform of the 1920s now crystallized into a conservative ideological position. The AMA portrayed the CCMC's recommendations as "socialist dogma" (Stevens, 1971). Dr. Morris Fishbein, *Journal of the AMA* editor, led the attack on the CCMC majority report—and effectively killed it—in a *JAMA* editorial published just a few days after the report was publicly unveiled:

> Briefly, the majority report recommends that medical practice be rendered largely by organized groups associated with hospitals, and it expresses the hope that these groups will maintain the personal relationship so essential to good medical care. The rendering of all medical care by groups or guilds or medical Soviets has been one of the pet schemes of E.A. Filene.... The two reports [i.e. majority and minority] represent the difference between incitement to revolution and a desire for gradual evolution based on analysis and study.... The minority is willing to test any plan that may be offered if it conforms to the medical conception of what is known to be good medical practice.... The physicians of this country must not be misled by utopian fantasies of a form of medical practice which would equalize all physicians by placing them in groups under one administration.... It is better for the American people that most of their illnesses by treated by their own doctors rather than by industries, corporations or clinics. (Fishbein, 1932, pp. 1950–52)

The AMA in this editorial made the standard judgment of a utopia by a representative of a group in power: it is the unrealizable. At best this is a self-deceptive ignorance by that class, because the utopia may well be, what Ricoeur (1986) called a "relative utopia unrealizable only within the given order" (p. 177). Moreover, in this editorial, Fishbein implicitly framed the issue as "Americanism" vs. "Sovietism" (Walker, 1979). At the level of ideology as distortion, Fishbein's "Americanism" ideology was a ploy to hide the harsh reality that in the 1930s many workers were having trouble paying their hospital bills and many Americans did not have a personal physician. Fishbein's rhetoric of voluntarism was "an organizational ideology" (Rogin, 1959; 1962) that functioned to protect the social status quo and the established groups holding power in American medicine. A week later in another Fishbein editorial, this ideology became explicit: "There is moreover, a far greater concern that the rights of the physician to practice...There is the question of Americanism versus Sovietism for the American people" (quoted in Walker, 1979, p. 489). The issue of cost and access were cloaked under the labels of "Americanism" and the "sacred trust."

In terms of conceptual distortion and the use of established authority, Fishbein's work was brilliant. By naming the common enemy—"Sovietism"—he was able to hide the practitioner-academic split within medicine. This gave the illusion of a united medical coalition and created an appearance of power that attracted further allies such as the AHA (Fox 1986; Stevens 1989). "Americanism" also provided a positive symbolic sense of social identity, something needed in the Depression turmoil-policy as perspective. Edward Bernays, the CCMC majority's public relations man, warned them that Fishbein's editorial was a political hatchet job. He advised a public relations counterattack—something Franklin would have approved—but they put their trust in rational discourse and discussion (Walker, 1979). They rejected a policy strategy that would use public relations to arouse public passion for their proposal.

Fishbein defended the editorial as "an act in keeping with the best of American journalism" (quoted in Walker, 1979, p. 499). Years later, Fishbein inadvertently revealed, in another context, what he meant about journalism. In 1970, CBS ran a one-hour television documentary that was critical of the American health care system and the AMA's defense of the status quo. Fishbein wrote a letter to CBS criticizing its journalism which he charged aroused public passions, failed to mention certain facts, and generally was sensationalistic in approach. He wrote that people who understand American journalism know "how a story or news report can be slanted. By accumulating reports of dramatic incidents and publishing them all at one time, the public can be alarmed and be made to think in terms of an epidemic of such incidents" (Schorr, 1970, p. 207).

This is precisely the type of journalism Fishbein used in his 1932 editorial. This editorial failed to show that the minority report agreed with several majority report recommendations. This is a crucial inconvenient fact left unmentioned. Walker suggests that both reports "believed that the nation was far too complex for any [one] *plan* to succeed" (1979, p. 496–97, italics added), that is, the majority recommendations were not a master plan—were not a utopian fantasy. Moreover, Fishbein lumped together fact and fiction to warn the American public of a Communist conspiracy to collectivize its health care system: "The rendering of all medical care by groups or guilds or medical soviets has been one of the pet schemes of E.A. Filene, who probably was chiefly responsible for establishing the CCMC and in developing funds for its promotion." Now, while it is true that Filene, the Boston department store mogul, championed "medical guilds," he did not advocate "medical soviets." Indeed, "auto care," not dialectical materialism, was Filene's model. He advocated the application of scientific management to make health care more businesslike (Filene, 1929). By adding the fictitious "medical soviets," Fishbein aroused public fears of a communist takeover. He succeeded in framing the CCMC report in terms of ideological ideas such as "Americanism vs. Sovietism" (Walker, 1979).

Still, it is important to understand the healthy utopian aspect of the CCMC majority report. One of the research staff's leaders, on looking back, insisted that the majority report's "recommendations were primarily on what needed to be done toward the future of medicine through voluntary activities" (Falk, 1984, p. 26). Unfortunately, this voluntarism— as social learning—was not effectively communicated by the report's rhetoric. The radical utopian rhetoric of "cultural lag" dominated the text.

Interestingly, the *New York Times* analysis of the CCMC report picked up the cultural lag metaphor (Duffus, December 4, 1932). The *Times'* overall analysis pictures the policy debate as a clash of European social philosophies: socialization vs. individualism. However, in the section on individualism, the analyst stressed the extent to which the laity would under the majority report's recommendations have a voice in determining medical care public policy. This is the earlier Franklinian theme of community participation. This was suppressed as the AMA succeeded in framing the issue written in the European polarity: "socialism vs. individualism."

The CCMC majority report can, I believe, be usefully redescribed— in Deweyan terms (1894) it can be "set free from its local and partial bonds"—as a pragmatic approach stressing the need for community action to explore local American health care possibilities. In a sense, this pragmatic strand was a hidden, second minority report. In its introduction to the report's recommendations, the Committee stressed an experimental, incremental pace. It was against a dogmatic and revolutionary tempo of change. It emphasized that medical system problems would vary from region to region and therefore no panacea could exist, no single solution would be appropriate for all these various regions. While offering a comprehensive vision, it urged incremental experimentation. Rather than offering a single solve-all-problems plan, it called for adapting general principles to local situations. It advocated local control and responsiveness and argued against excessive centralization. And it stressed that the incremental process might take thirty years to complete. It grew out of the social survey tradition (CCMC, 1932, pp. 104–8).

> Fortunately, we have retained in this country, a wholesome *local responsibility* for medical services. This means that *opportunities* exist for trying out many plans under various and variable conditions. Where action can be limited to the city or county, we have thousands of *experiment* stations.... The Committee urges the broadest sympathy toward *experimentation* in promising fields, together with the most searching analysis of the results (CCMC, 1932, p. 108, italics added). There is a growing conviction that social evolution may be guided wisely and that it is *statesmanlike* to formulate the objectives of such evolution. What is true of society is true of medical service, for as long as society is on the march, medical service will inevitably be on the march too, and should have a clear vision of the goal ahead (CCMC, p. 58, italics added). European countries may not have proceeded with the greatest wisdom, but they have acted (CCMC, p. 149. italics added).

Interestingly, for each of the "three lines of approach" that the majority report recommends, it provided for considerable flexibility. First, hospitals, medical groups or industrial medical services could become a hub of a regionally organized system. Second, group prepayment could be public or private. Third, a period of local experimentation was urged. A specific approach would be tailored to fit community type, the socioeconomic group to be served and the services to be provided. Regional health planning agencies could be funded by a variety of voluntary organizations, be led by local physicians, but include a variety of local lay people and could well grow out of existing agencies. The recommendations were healthy utopian projections of actual existing examples with "community" as a basic consideration. Essentially, the cultural lag here became an *organizational gap* that could be closed by physician/expert and community cooperation. Polarization implied by the "lag" metaphor is replaced by the "gaps" invitation for participation.

Fox argues that the CCMC advocates for a regional approach to health care planning had "universalism" as their goal, that is, they stressed the need to have medical services of uniform quality uniformly available throughout a region (1986, p. 19). He contrasts this with the "particularate" orientation of economic development regionalists whose aim was stimulating economic growth and making an area more livable. Since the CCMC was in part action-oriented and focused on regional, not national approaches and standards, the recommendations quoted above strike me as not universalistic, but particularistic. In Deweyan terms, the recommendations are presented as a prod to community adaptation: "These recommendations are flexible and *adaptable*. But they do not exhaust the possibilities. The future is pregnant with opportunity. The *local community* must determine through careful study what kind of program is best adapted to its own *particular* needs" (CCMC, p. 148, italics added).

Moreover, some CCMC staffers were clearly particularists. Rufus Rorem, who helped write the report, went on to foster the local-based Blue Cross movement and later the regional health planning movement (McNerney, 1982; Sigmond, 1982). Recently, Fox described Rorem and his fellow early Blue Cross pioneers as "intensely pragmatic" (1993, p. 93). Rorem was a "practical visionary" (Sigmond, 1982, p. 59). As for group practice and group payment, he "accepted either separately or in any order. He saw group financing and delivery as a means to the end, to the goal of...predictability, and he was flexible regarding means" (McNerney, 1982, xxl). It was this flexibility that would give local communities room to maneuver as they might try to work out local application to general policy recommendations. Rorem had a faith in local voluntary leadership to explore the possible. He thought that eventually group practice and group payment would be conjoined (Sigmond, 1982, p. 60). Interestingly, while Rorem was a progressive in his personal notion of consumerism as represented by a community's established leaders, the CCMC's flexible recommendation of medical center governance at least had an open door to more populist forms—as long as they were effective. Rorem's particularist, social learning perspective could be seen in his position in the 1930s against merging local Blue Cross Plans into statewide corporations. He had his eye on the community (McNerney, 1982).

The CCMC was part of the social survey movement. Within this sociological movement there were concepts that were not, Janowitz (1978) observed, easily combined. For example, Ogburn's theory of "cultural lag" offered a mechanical deterministic picture of society driven forward by technology, leaving obsolete traditions, and so on behind. This pointed back towards universalistic planning. On the other hand, some sociologists were putting forth a theory of social assimilation in which old, primordial attachments would be carried forward into new social arrangements. These sociologists believed that such attachments would neither disappear nor survive unchanged, but rather would be attenuated and provide a basis for new arrangements. They emphasized the role of voluntary associations (Janowitz, 1978). The CCMC majority report followed this second, social learning perspective when it envisioned carrying forward the patient-doctor traditional relationship, but within a new, more formally structured social-organizational context. Lewis Mumford's writing at the time illustrates what the CCMC process looks like seen through a progressive lens. For him regional planning was a participatory, democratic process of social learning that used surveys to establish facts and motivate citizens to see their region in terms of a workable utopian vision (Friedmann, 1987).

The CCMC's majority report has been a reference point in American health policy debate for sixty years now. Dr. Fishbein's rhetorical success has lingered for decades. The "cultural lag" advocates succeeded in presenting themselves as noble victims (Fox, 1986). The majority report and its reception unproductively led to decades of ideological "Americanism vs. Sovietism" framed debate which helped preserve the status quo (Walker, 1977; Fox, 1986). Still, the report also was a utopian prod to health care change. As Walker suggests, the report "represented the beginning of a transition in thought regarding ways to improve and extend health care" (Walker, 1979, p. 504).

Blue Cross (1929–1960)

The Blue Cross and Blue Shield movements were mid-twentieth century success stories (while the separate prepaid group practice movement was a social experiment that refused to fold in the face of organized medicine's opposition). The first Blue Cross Plan was started in Dallas, Texas in 1929 with 1000 enrollees (Anderson, 1975). The percentage of the U.S. population covered by health insurance was less than two percent in 1930 and half a century later had risen to 82 percent. The Blues spearheaded this achievement. Meanwhile, many consumer-governed HMOs trace their movement back to 1927 and the cooperative prepaid group practice started by Dr. Michael Shadid in Elk City, Oklahoma. Today's Kaiser-Permanent program traces its history back to 1933. In general, prepaid group practice—another CCMC recommendation—struggled to establish a beachhead in various American communities (Anderson, 1985).

In the early 1930s, the Rosenwald Fund (which had helped fund the CCMC) decided to get out of medical care research because of medical opposition (Anderson, 1975). It gave Rorem, who had been on its medical research staff before he left to work for the CCMC, guardianship over $100,000 to give to some worthy nonprofit agency of his own selection. Rorem invested the funds in building a new agency to promote hospital group prepayment. This project was to evolve into the Blue Cross movement (Anderson, 1975).

There are some connections between Rosenwald, Rorem, Dewey, and Benjamin Franklin. First, as Boorstin (1987) has observed, Rosenwald and Franklin both shared the same conception of philanthropy as a public process of community institution building, and not private individual acts of charity. Drucker (1987) suggests that what made Rosenwald innovative was his interest in building—that is, empowering—both citizens and their communities. Rosenwald, like Franklin and Dewey, focused on encouraging practical habits and skills to increase citizen and community self-reliance and capability. He funded the county farm agent and 4-H Club movements. It makes sense then that Rorem's Blue Cross activity should be funded by Rosenwald's foundation. Both of them were interested in institution building, in forwarding self-help and community capability. Also, Rosenwald was against self-perpetuating foundations. His fund was to exist for only twenty-five years and then go out of business. He felt that foundations' objectives were contingent, context-bound, and hence bound to become outmoded. This brings to mind Dewey's opposition to the idea of fixed, external, ends-in-themselves. He saw only temporarily useful ends-in-views. Such a distinction was at the heart of Rosenwald's position on this issue. Instead of a false quest for certainty, Rosenwald was prepared to take risks in the pursuit of ends-in-view.

Rorem also shares a family resemblance with Dewey. Rorem was able to see what was distinctive and doable in a situation—what Adams called a meroscopic perspective. Hospital prepayment was for Rorem pivotal. As he recalled "From my point of view we had picked the key point where all the conflicts and changes were going to come" (Anderson, 1975, p. 30). He actually had a keener personal interest in group practice, but saw that hospital prepayment was what the situation called for and would permit (Sigmond, 1990). His attitude was nondoctrinaire. He once said, "In the field at the time I was thought of as a safe man. Mike Davis was considered dangerous by organized medicine. As a matter of fact, I was probably more radical in many respects" (Anderson, 1975, p. 37). Like Franklin, then, Rorem's quiet, conciliatory style hid a challenge to the status quo.

Rorem regarded the CCMC's radical ideas such as group practice, regional health planning, and group prepayment as means (i.e., ends-in-view) and not ends-in-themselves. As such he readily unbundled them and pursued the one that was doable in the prevailing circumstances of the 1930s. He could look at a set of proposed ideas and select the doable elements for piecemeal reform. It was this imaginative flexibility that let him also create Blue Cross' flexible guidelines that were useful in giving the movement some discipline, while allowing them to be adaptable to unique local settings (McNerney, 1982). Rorem was "a practical visionary" who pursued "here and now objectives" within a long-term perspective (Sigmond, 1982, p. 59). As Robert Sigmond said of his long-term colleague and friend: "Dr. Rorem was always more interested in getting something done than in getting something perfect, but he never worked in a narrow perspective" (p. 60). He was interested in utopian institution building that was presently realizable.

This recalls Dewey's distinction between declaring that something is "satisfying" vs. "satisfactory." "Satisfying" is what management theorists call "satisfycing," which is a response to a problem that is merely "good enough," something that is an immediate stopgap. "Satisfactory," on the other hand, involves an act of practical judgment that makes the best of a given situation. A satisfactory response is judged in terms of both its immediate and future consequences (Dewey, 1955). Rorem always tried to find things that were "satisfactory." This anticipated Selznick's view of creative leadership (1983).

Light (1991) captures the Franklin-like qualities of Rorem: his conciliatory posture and his ability to invent an institution into place:

> [It] was the soft-spoken, self-effacing Quaker, C. Rufus Rorem, and a small group of colleagues who realized that a prepaid hospital plan would have to include many or all of the hospitals in an area so that the doctor and the patient could have free choice.... The genius of Rorem's vision lay in persuading state legislatures that in lieu of the sizable reserves required of insurance plans, hospitals could substitute guaranteed services. Indeed, *the trick* of early multi-hospital plan administrators was to negotiate a contract of payments with hospitals for their services that lay within the limits of the $.50/$1.00 per month that subscribers were willing to pay in. (Light, 1991, p. 56, italics added)

Rorem's trick was even more elegant. Hospitals in the Depression already were losing money on patients who could not pay their bills.

Hospitals, therefore, had nothing further to lose by underwriting with their services Blue Cross Plan's financial risk—and much to gain. Rorem had combined public and private in inventing Blue Cross prepayment much as Franklin had with his matching grant fund raising scheme. Rorem was a health care political educator and intellectual midwife to the Blue Cross movement.

Rorem, in Deweyan terms, pursued ends-in-view with an eye to long-term consequences. But the meaning of consequences depends on what basic considerations inform one's social imagination. What were Rorem's considerations? A provocative hint is provided by the title he gave to a collection of his papers and articles: *A Quest for Certainty* (1982). Dewey's *The Quest for Certainty* (1929) argued against the search for certainties, against "ends-in-themselves." As Dewey wrote elsewhere: "Love of certainty is a demand for guarantees in advance of action. Ignoring the fact that truth can be bought only by the adventure of experiment, dogmatism turns truth into an insurance company" (1964). Dewey rejected the quest for ideological or utopian certitude. He urged innovation. In this light, Rorem's title is ironic: we have myths that provisionally impassion us with a useful illusion of certitude. As Sigmond observed about Rorem: "Certainty was the Holy Grail—the unobtainable. Self-interest is central in America, combined with some degree of community service" (1990). Translating this into Deweyan terms, "Community" was Rorem's compass point as America traveled on its endless quest for "certainty." "Community" was the radical idea that Rorem the progressive strove to stamp into Blue Cross' character. The utopian "community" helped him as a statesperson see that one era's false (actually provisional) health care end-in-itself is actually a contingent end-in-view. As McNerney (1982) noted about Rorem's book title, it shows that today's problem is not just cost containment, but rather cost containment-quality-access, and so on.

The government, according to Rorem, stresses equity and certainty, while the private sector can emphasize experimentation and innovation (Anderson, 1975). Here Rorem followed Franklin and Dewey by avoiding a structural "individual versus society" distinction, instead he used the public/private functional distinction of Dewey. Dewey stressed that it was useful to remember that the private sector was good at innovation and experiment, while the public sector was reliable with respect to routine matters (1976). Rorem, then, looked at Blue Cross as an experiment in how to voluntarily bring health care coverage to American wage earn-ers (Hedinger, 1968; Brown, 1991a).

Of the thirty-nine Blue Cross plans started in the 1930s about half got their start-up funds exclusively from hospitals, half from a variety of local community sources (Law, 1974). Most treatments of Blue Cross origins (e.g., Light, 1991; Starr, 1982) stress a "sin of commission": the co-optation of the Blue Cross movement by the hospital field. Complementing this was, however, a "sin of omission": the failure of the Community Chest and Coun-cils of America to sponsor Rorem and his Blue Cross activity (Anderson, 1975). Rorem went first to the Community Chest and Councils, but they rejected Rorem's Blue Cross project because it did not meet their rigid—un-Franklinian—definition of charity. Like Franklin, Rorem had to rein-vent his innovation by means of coalition building. Had the Blue Cross movement been under Community Chest auspices, or been able to be housed at the Rosenwald Fund, the prepayment experiment might well have leaned farther in the direction of a destiny marked by democratic participation and regional development.

From the start there was a tension in the Blue Cross movement be-tween its leadership—headed by the brilliantly conciliatory Rufus Rorem—and the vast majority of Blue Cross Plan directors who were more conservative. The leadership saw Blue Cross as a community ser-vice agency, as a form of social insurance. Most Plan executives, how-ever, saw it more as an insurance company that was a financing agency for hospitals (Anderson, 1975; Law, 1974). So, Blue Cross' character has always been ambivalent, combining elements of commercial ideology with those of communitarian utopianism. All, however, saw the value of a community image. Blue Cross adapted the language of community-minded consumer cooperatives. Salesmen were called "representatives," customers were called "members," and so on (Anderson, 1975). In the 1930s Rorem and others were able to get virtually all states to pass spe-cial enabling legislation tailor-made for establishing Blue Cross Plans. At the same time organized medicine was succeeding in many states in getting legislation passed that made prepaid group practices illegal.

In the 1940s the Blues' growth continued, although many physicians feared that someday, the Blues would achieve an independent power-base and reorganize the American delivery system (Stevens, 1989). Despite such misgivings, the AMA ran advertisements after World War II for the Blues as a tactic to discourage the coming of either national health insurance or prepaid group practice (Stevens, 1989). One upshot of World War II was that health insurance became an attractive collective bargaining benefit (Anderson, 1985; Stevens, 1989). Another upshot of the war was that many young physicians had been favorable impressed by their experience with group practice while in the armed forces. This would spur the growth in group practice when they returned to civilian life (Fox, 1986).

While providers feared that Blue Cross would grow too powerful, the local Blue Cross Plans themselves actually resisted moves in that direction. Throughout the 1940s, John Mannix, of the Cleveland Plan, was a Blue Cross movement "gadfly" (Anderson, 1975, p. 50), prodding his fellow Blue Cross executive directors to establish a national mechanism for marketing Blue Cross to nationwide employers. Mannix had a "lone and swashbuckling style" (Anderson, 1975, p. 51) that put him too far ahead of his more conservative colleagues. His radical centralizing business idea was rejected and his fellow Blue Cross CEOs saw him at times a "dangerous man," to borrow Rorem's terminology. He threatened their local autonomy and self-interest.

In 1944 Mannix proposed establishing, under a federal charter, an "American Blue Cross" that would have carried basic principles like not-for-profit orientation, community rating, and so on. forward to meet national account needs. It would also have offered a comprehensive medical-hospital set of benefits. Essentially, he argued that the idea of local voluntarism could only progress by means of effective nationwide mechanisms (Mannix, 1944).

Meanwhile, in the 1940s prepaid group practices arrived as collective bargaining options in a handful of cities around the nation. They were emerging as a yardstick to measure affordable health care (Anderson, 1985). After the war, Henry J. Kaiser publicly debated Morris Fishbein on health care reform, contributing to Fishbein's fall from AMA power (Foster, 1990). In part offering health care fringe benefits to workers was a way of buying domestic tranquillity after the war (Navarro, 1990; Nisbet, 1988). The auto industry, for example, was making record-breaking profits by selling cars to the rapidly growing middle class. It gave its workers large wage increases and health benefits. It then passed the cost along to the customer. This disturbed Walter Reuther, UAW President (Halberstam, 1986).

In the 1950s, Blue Cross enrollment growth slowed as commercial insurers entered the market. Blue Shield growth, meanwhile, increased. Health care costs and Blue Cross rates began to escalate (Anderson, 1975;

1985). As Blue Cross premiums escalated, unions began to become concerned with medical care costs (Fox, 1986). A few progressive unions reacted to this problem by becoming involved with prepaid group practice initiatives (Starr, 1982). These union leaders were joined by other community leaders in a movement for reforming local health care systems. The medical and business worlds had still not accepted prepaid group practice's legitimacy. David Stewart, Rochester, New York, Blue Cross executive director from the 1950s through the early 1980s, recalls some community health political dynamics:

> One of the problems we had is that the Captains of Industry were greatly influenced by the physicians with whom they played golf and associated with at the country club. I would go on a campaign to try to persuade a local Captain of Industry on some course of action and then he would go play golf with some eminent surgeon friend of his and by Monday I was further back than when I first started. This happened all over the country (Stewart, 1990).

Also, when the 1950s started, Stewart (1990) recalls that many Blue Shield Plans with their own physician-composed boards, shared the local Blue Cross Plan's director. As Blue Shield enrollment increased, the rising physician feeling was that Blue Cross was too liberal and not protective enough of the medical community. This led to some of these Blue Shield Plans splitting off from Blue Cross management in order to have more control of management. Blue Cross executive directors who wanted to keep their Blue Shield Plans from splitting off had to avoid talking about reform ideas like prepaid group practice (Stewart, 1990). This led to the 1950s being a time of deep acrimony at the local level between reformers and organized medicine which was not ready for reform. For the most part, prepaid group practice activity was frustrated (Stevens, 1989).

Meanwhile, Blue Cross tried to meet the commercials' invasion by adopting their rival's methods such as experience rating which broke down the community's overall risk pool and gave relatively healthier employee groups lower rates based on the group's actual experience in service usage. As Blue Cross critic Sylvia Law (1974) observes, Blue Cross did not have a choice in adopting experience rating methods if it hoped to compete with its commercial rivals. This bothered the Blue Cross movement's moral leadership. James Stuart, chairman of the Blue Cross Commission, wrote a widely read article in *Modern Hospital* in which he protested the degradation of Blue Cross' community service ideal in the 1950s; he lamented the gap between the Blue Cross ideal and its commercial practices:

> We found ourselves thinking and spending in insurance terms, and in some areas using the methods, technics and concepts of traditional commercial insurance. If our function is simply to provide hospital insurance...we should...throw off the cloak of community service and stand for what we are: 87 relatively small companies writing hospitalization insurance. (Quoted in Anderson, 1975, p. 67)

"Community" for Stuart was a utopian ideal that could be partially and meaningfully realized; he resented its conversion into a mere ideological ploy. This ploy marked the beginning of the end of Blue Cross as a social movement. As Blue Cross rate increases escalated in the 1950s around the country, the handful of internal Blue Cross critics were joined by mounting public criticism. Also in the 1950s, the leadership of the loose Blue Cross confederation began to consider, for practical business reasons, establishing some mechanism to market to national accounts (Anderson, 1975). In general, the 1945–1960 period of Blue Cross evolution was one in which the Blue Cross plans for the most part refused to take in the meaning of the past, nor did they turn to the future. Insiders report that the plans were overly cautious and not ready for the challenge (Mannix, 1959), academic observers see it as a drift into "dogmatic privatism" (Brown, 1991b, p. 658).

The national health policy situation was, on the other, hand, relatively tranquil. It was the Eisenhower years in which growth and increased access was the strategy for dealing with social problems (Starr, 1982). Efforts to pass legislation that might provide funds to cover the capital and start-up costs for developing prepaid group practices were defeated (Starr, 1982; Stevens, 1971). At the same time the AMA's Larson Report (AMA, 1959) accepted prepaid group practice as a legitimate alternate delivery system. The 1950s were also in some ways years of wastefulness. For example, G.M. took the newly invented high compression engine—intended to improve auto fuel efficiency—and used it to build gas guzzlers. When Reuther complained, the auto leaders replied that they had to build the highly profitable big cars, in part, to pay for their employees' lavish fringe benefits, which included Blue Cross and Blue Shield coverage (Halberstam, 1986).

The CCMC report was about right, the incremental development of Blue Cross, one of its key recommendations, took about thirty years (1929–1960) to approach maturity. This offers some time perspective to the next thirty-five years (1960–1995) as the loose Blue Cross confederation's HMO involvement slowly evolved from parochial ignorance to nationwide marketing and managed care. Drucker (1987) sums up the managerial lesson about institution building from Rosenwald's social learning experience. Drucker emphasizes the need for time to build up a fund of appropriate skills for the job. He observes that for a social program to do anything beyond consume a lot of money, time is needed to slowly build up a cadre of distinctively competent people. He goes on:

> First rate people are always in short supply.... The growth curve of social programs is the hyperbola; very small, almost imperceptible results for long hard years followed, if the program is successful, by years of exponential growth.... [L]earning has a long lead time before it shows massive results. Individuals, not classes, learn; and there has to be built up, one by one, a large stock of individuals who have learned, who serve as examples, as multipliers, as leaders, and who give encouragement. (1987, p. 145)

Hence, social learning, the key to institution building, has a long lead time. Short-term policy evaluation is, therefore, often misguided and counter-productive, especially if it judges an experiment's immediate modest consequences in terms of grandiose antecedent goals. Institution building on a nationwide scale is a slow process because it requires accumulating a "distinctive competence" (Selznick, 1983, p. 53).

The early Blue Cross experiment succeeded in that it demonstrated the practicality of health insurance. It also brought its own new problems. How would the Blues respond to the critical challenge of the commercials, government and emerging community needs? Could new life be infused into the Blue Cross concept? Could the institution be reconstructed to meet the needs of a new situation?

2

Exhortation About A Radical Idea (1960s)

As we turn to an interpretation of Blue Cross HMO institution building across a thirty-five year period, it is useful to recall Selznick's point
that leadership involves: "creation of conditions that will make possible
in the future what is excluded in the present" (1983, p. 154). For Blue
Cross Association HMO building this involved three steps. Indiana University basketball coach Robert Knight's notion of strategic positioning
provides a useful clue to such steps. Feinstein (1986) describes Knight
talking to his team early in an Indiana basketball season this way: "We
are now 2-2 in the Big Ten.... We have three home games coming up—
Ohio State, Purdue, Illinois. We have now put ourselves into a position
where, if we can win these three games, we'll be in a position to be a
factor in the Big Ten race" (p. 193). In the agitated 1960s McNerney ex-
pounded upon the radical prepaid group practice concept. He took the
Blue Cross confederation from non-HMO involvement to initial consideration by a few Blue Cross Plans—the equivalent of being 2 and 2 at the
start of the Big Ten basketball season. This set the stage for the 1970s
where some Blue Cross Plans experimented with HMOs (like winning
the next three Big Ten games). This established the Blues in a position to
be a factor in the national HMO competition of the 1980s and 1990s.
(McNerney resigned in 1981 and was succeeded by Bernard Tresnowski
who in turn retired in 1994). In the 1980s many Blue Cross Plans had
HMOs and most of these HMOs succeeded in the market place. Today,
the Blue Cross and Blue Shield confederation ranks first nationally in
terms of total HMO enrollment, and has more HMOs in more states than
any other entry in the market. As one former Blue Cross Association HMO
staffer recalls: "In terms of the Blue Cross [Association's HMO effort] it
got in early and started to *talk the subject* and educated some folks, then
it *threw a little money* at it and waited for the *marketplace to react* one

way or the other and when it did, Blue Cross was in a position to develop businesses that responded to the demand."

The Blues Get a Statesman:
Institution Building Leadership As A Rhetorical Art

In 1961 the young and small Blue Cross Association (BCA) recruited Walter J. McNerney, a former hospital manager, as its new president. In some important ways this selection was shaped by two events of 1955 and their aftermath. The first dealt with Blue Cross' efficacy as a community service organization; the second with its capacity to serve national accounts. In short, the dual shadows of Rorem and Mannix. First, in 1955 the Blue Cross Plan in Michigan announced a then unheard of 20 percent rate increase which was met by a state government call for an investigation. This then took the form of a foundation-funded, comprehensive health services research survey of health care delivery and financing in Michigan. This was the most comprehensive health care study since the Committee on the Costs of Medical Care. The study team was assembled and directed by the thirty-two-year-old director of the University of Michigan's health services administration department, Walter J. McNerney.

The second event was the dozen largest Blue Cross plans (which combined had one half of the total Blue Cross enrollment nationwide) holding a secret meeting in New York City to explore ways to tackle a marketing problem. Local Blue Cross enrollment growth was slowing in the face of rising commercial insurance competition. The proposed solution was to use the fledgling Blue Cross Association (which unlike the Blue Cross Commission was not a unit of the American Hospital Association) as a vehicle to market Blue Cross policies to national accounts. The reason for the secrecy was that the self-proclaimed "Millionaires Club" (those Plans that each had at least a million subscribers) did not intend to let the other sixty-five Blue Cross plans' foot-dragging slow or veto the national account marketing initiative (Anderson, 1975). When this marketing effort subsequently faltered, James Stuart (Cincinnati Blue Cross president) came in to head BCA. In 1959 he suggested that the AHA-based Blue Cross Commission had outlived its usefulness and that there should be just one agency, the independent Blue Cross Association (BCA). Despite the misgivings of many plan CEOs that BCA would create an overly centralized system that could control the Plans, Stuart's idea was accepted. Nonetheless, the BCA's national account initiative failed (Anderson, 1975).

As Stuart, the Blue Cross movement's moral conscience in the 1950s, looked forward towards retirement, the search for a successor began. The Blue Cross confederation's progressive leaders—about a half-dozen in number—sought a relatively young, nonideological leader who, Anderson suggests, "was not associated with past prejudices and vested interests among plan directors. Instead an outsider was sought" (Anderson, 1975, p. 83). McNerney was selected. It should be noted that some progressive plan directors backed Thomas Tierney, the young innovative Colorado Plan director, for the position. These directors favored someone who was already in the business (Stewart, 1990). However, Stuart and McNary of the Michigan Plan successfully pushed McNerney's candidacy.

As an outsider, McNerney was a bit like Franklin in Philadelphia: a stranger with strong degrees of freedom with respect to his new environment. Crucially, McNerney was selected for his political and rhetorical skills. Richard Brockway, (Massachusetts Plan director at the time and on the search committee) recalls that McNerney had combined academic and medical care political experience in Michigan. What impressed people were his public communication skills. Brockway recalls: "My fondest memory is that when we were considering McNerney and I didn't know a thing about him, I called a professor I knew well at the University of Michigan. I asked him what he knew about McNerney. He said, "He's very conservative. You don't want to have him around." So I said, "Look, how is he in relation to the medical field?" And he said, "Oh, he's a flaming radical!" (Brockway, 1990). From the perspective of utopia as magical radical thought, McNerney was conservative. From the perspective of ideology as preservation of the medical status quo he was radical.

The search committee was looking for someone who could preserve Blue Cross' identity by prodding it into a constructive future. In 1959 three Blue Cross leaders wrote separate articles that reveal what they were looking for in national association leadership: concern for preserving the community service identity of Blue Cross, turning it away from being a financial arm of hospitals to being the public means for controlling costs, better serving national accounts (Stuart, McNary & Mannix, 1959). McNerney's intention was to, in Stevens' words, "strengthen the authority of Blue Cross interests, nationally, in negotiations with the federal government, and as a power able to deal with the insurance industry, and also to develop the association as an organization that would be closer to hospitals at the national level" (Stevens, 1989, p. 265). She goes on to note that an initial step that McNerney took was a federally funded research project investigating federal worker's hospital utilization rates, comparing those in a prepaid group practice with those in the traditional fee-for-service, Blue Cross system. She observes that such hospital utilization studies done in that period indicated considerable waste; that is, unnecessary hospitalization in the traditional system.

Such a study would, however, give credence to the feeling, growing since 1955, that doctors and hospitals—health care's established powers—were potential exploiters of hospitalization (Stevens, 1989, p. 265). Thus, it would not serve McNerney's stated intention of BCA working closer with the American Hospital Association (AHA). The proposed study was a challenge to the health care establishment and was therefore politically explosive. Therefore, McNerney did not propose the study until 1967 and it was rejected for funding by the Public Health Service in 1968. It was subsequently funded in 1970, with its initial results published in 1975. (Later a second report came out in book form in 1984.) In short, it took McNerney ten years to propose and get the study funded. Health care politics had allowed no greater speed.

The key to understanding McNerney's handling of the prepaid group practice research idea lies in his leadership style. To understand this it will be useful to look at some seminal and relevant books on leadership in the 1950s and 1960s. Gardner's *Self-Renewal* (1963) warned against organizational dry rot, rigidity, and vested interests. He called for nationwide organizational renewal and challenge to the status quo—guided by a moral purpose. He wrote: "Experienced...managers know that some organizations can be renewed through new leadership and new ideas. Others need a more massive infusion of new blood or far-reaching organizational changes" (1963, p. 76).

Gardner's thoughts nicely summarize the BCA search committee's concern about vested interests and the need for leadership. These reflections also raise the question of what new ideas, organizational changes and new blood McNerney would be injecting into the Blue Cross confederation. And this raises the general issues of organizational renewal. Today, some of our best organization theorists (e.g., Wilson, *Bureaucracy*, 1990) are focusing once again on organizational purpose, mission, and beliefs. Still, the emphasis is on, as it was with Selznick in 1957, preserving established organizations and not with renewal or innovation. As Starr notes there is a need to understand what "leadership can do today to create the sense of purpose and commitment that has been so crucial to the most successful agencies" (Starr, 1990, p. 41).

Although most of Selznick's work deals with the conservative task of institutional survival, and not enough with creative response to environmental changes, it ends with some reflections on creative leadership, change and reconstruction. The creative leader, the statesperson must, Selznick argues, embody the institution's purpose, that is, its mission. This mission must respond to the leader's strategic analysis of the environment. The leader has to transform men and women into participants in the institution's purpose. In this educational process, the effective leader is a communicator who interprets the organization's mission, character and role. The statesman is a political educator. One effective way to infuse institutional life with purpose and meaning, Selznick suggests, is the creation of realizable utopian visions. Selznick writes:

> These are efforts to state, in the language of uplift and idealism, what is distinctive about the aims and methods of the enterprise.... Myths are institution builders.... The art of the creative leader is the art of institution building, the reworking of human and technological materials to fashion an organism that embodies new and enduring values. The opportunity to do this depends on a considerable sensitivity to the politics of change.... One great leadership function is the creation of conditions that will make possible in the future what is excluded in the present. This requires a strategy of change that looks to the attainment of new capabilities more nearly fulfilling the truly felt needs and aspirations of the institution. The executive becomes a statesman as he makes the transition from administrative management to institutional leadership. (1983, pp. 153–54)

A creative statesman, then, uses rhetoric to mediate change and thereby rebuilds an institution.

The BCA selection criteria for its new president involved many of Gardner and Selznick's points. The search committee was concerned with both immediate political and market pressures and with preserving or renewing Blue Cross' community-focused identity. There was concern about the dry rot of vested interests in the Blue Cross confederation—and the expedient adoption of commercial insurer methods which eroded Blue Cross principles. A new leader with new ideas was sought, but there were some understandable misgivings about an academician's potential for utopian flights of fancy. Also, although Plan executives saw a need for organizational changes, most feared BCA ploys, feared it would become too power seeking. They strongly resisted centralization. They sought a leader who would have political savvy and communications skills, as well as a vision of how American health care could evolve.

When the BCA search committee selected McNerney, they did not know yet the specifics of how he saw Blue Cross' mission, role, distinctive competence, and so on. The educational process of mythmaking lay ahead. Still, there was an irony involved in the search committee's decision that they did not need an elder statesman, but rather a relatively young person who would have the time to shape the confederation over a span of years. The irony is this: they selected a young statesman. And any statesperson in Selznick's view, transcends his or her specialism. McNerney recalls, in Selznickian terms concerning self-concept: "I never thought totally as a Blue Cross person. I saw my role in life as a statesman in the health field, of which Blue Cross was a part. I was equally anxious to have doctors and hospitals upgrade their vision and community orientation, as I was concerned with working out good ways to pay for things through the financing mechanism (McNerney, 1990).

McNerney was there to reconstruct Blue Cross. Leadership, for McNerney, involves getting others to think in a larger framework, one that reveals the fuller potential of situations. For example, for him the job of university programs in health administration is to inject into the healthcare field "gadflies, provocateurs" who would prod their organizations to see the larger picture (McNerney, 1984). When BCA recruited the director of the Michigan health administration program, they were making just such a pragmatic gadfly their president. Notice that McNerney was out not only to adjust Blue Cross to its environment—but to change and reshape that environment. He wanted to not only rebuild Blue Cross organizations but to also remake the American institution of medical care.

He once favorably described another trade association as being "a critical force, acting as an educator, as a researcher, as a gadfly, as a communicator and as a clarifier of issues" (McNerney, 1979, p. 8). He urged the group to "stay on the high road of community needs." This brings to mind Selznick's stress on social renewal guided by some higher moral purpose. It is also a good description of how McNerney saw BCA under his command. This relates to a fundamental distinction in terms of leadership. Ricoeur (1986) distinguishes between the Socratic notion of being a gadfly of social change and the Weberian concept of being a charismatic leader. The first is a political educator; the second a savior. Moreover,

Ricoeur cautions that while the gadfly style risks an overestimation of the power of facts and persuasive discussion, the charismatic style risks ruinous flights of fancy. In a telling remark he made in his Blue Cross Association (BCA) annual report to the Plans in 1964 (Blue Cross Association, 1964), McNerney said that BCA had to show "intellectual leadership." He explained: "To put it succinctly, he who knows and communicates, controls." Organizational leadership is in part a contest of ideas (Pettigrew, 1987). Ideas, if rhetoric is used effectively, legitimate action. Knowing flows from research. Control for him was an art involving facts gained from research plus a balance of provider relations, political and negotiating skills, and sophisticated measures of performance.

"Communication" is an interesting term in his power equation of "Knowledge + Communication = Control." Here we can expand on Selznick's idea that institution building is a creative leadership art. Odin Anderson has characterized the American health care system as an "uneasy equilibrium." An organization, in Selznick's view, needs to interpret its mission and role in language that relates to the social system in which it is located. It follows, then, that a health care organization such as Blue Cross gets anxious when its social equilibrium gets more uneasy. It must develop and display a distinctive competence that aligns it with the community's currently perceived identity. This is a rhetorical task. Rhetoric is, to give a simple definition, the art of persuasive communication. "The speaker seeks to provide the audience with reasons for adopting a new attitude or taking a new course of action. In this sense, rhetoric is the art of shaping society, changing the course of individuals and communities, setting patterns for new action" (Buchanan, 1989, p. 93).

Renewal, then involves rhetoric. Blue Cross in needing to continually demonstrate to its relevant communities that it is indispensable "today" shares the rhetorical status of an artwork. Harold Rosenberg once said about an artwork: "Its nature is contingent upon recognition by the current communion of the knowing. Art does not exist. *It declares itself* " (quoted in Buchanan, 1989, p. 106). Put another way, an artwork has to declare its identity and persuade its audience to perceive it that way. For Blue Cross, an anxious organization, this means it has to persuade its relevant audiences that it is at different times, for example, "businesslike" or "community-oriented." McNerney, as an institutional statesman, was in important ways a rhetorical leader. McNerney characterizes what I am calling his pragmatism as something both necessary and risky: "You're missing the point if you use the word 'pragmatism' in the wrong sense. The key is having a vision. And the desire to pull it off.... [You need to know] the practical aspects of how you get it done. Do you throw yourself on the fire or have a sense of patience?" (1990). Here McNerney was advocating mediating between utopian ends and ideological means, a utopian vision for him was only useful if it was realizable. Hence it had to be tied to practical means and approached processually, that is, not all at once, but over time.

McNerney Shapes Blue Cross Language: Coming To Terms With Change (1961–1967)

In enlisting McNerney, the BCA search committee—which was made up of the confederation's most progressive members—were deliberately hiring a young leader—McNerney was thirty-six years old—who in Odin Anderson's words, would "live into the future and shape it" (1975, p. 83). There was recognition of the need for, in our terms, institution building. They saw that Blue Cross could not remain as merely the hospital's financing arm. Moving away from this focus would involve words and deeds. In terms of action McNerney moved on two fronts. First he strengthened the Blue Cross confederation's national operating base by, for example, adding staff and developing plan performance evaluation indictors. Second, he set up a committee to study the hot political issue of health insurance for the aged. This was part of the initial movement towards Medicare. Meanwhile he also rhetorically prepared the way for prepaid group practice research. His experiences with the Michigan health care study had taught him that when inquiry was on a potentially divisive topic, political leadership was required to pave the way, and to deal with antagonisms generated (McNerney, 1984).

In reviewing American health care in larger terms that stressed possibilities, McNerney arrived at BCA with a double-barreled vision of Blue Cross' role. They had to improve the efficiency of their traditional business and also offer new controls and alternatives: "This was a foreign language to the troops. I felt that way from day one, but didn't start talking about this till 1964—because it wasn't timely" (1990, pp. 1–2).

Crucial here is that Blue Cross Plans traditionally saw themselves as fiscal "pipelines" feeding hospitals (Blue Cross Association, 1971a, p. 16), whereas McNerney instead saw these intermediaries as something that could actively reshape other health care institutions in their environment. He was looking at Blue Cross from an institution building perspective—seeing institutions not as "conduits," but as active agents prodding their field into new forms and directions (Fuller, 1981). This was his "utopian vision." McNerney in the 1960s had an insight. As he recalled: "If you think about it, the self-fulfilling prophecy is a valid notion. You are what you think of yourself" (1984, p. 55). He believed that things could be as you envision them. As Stewart, his friend and former Blue Cross Plan president observes, McNerney's best tactic for influencing his board was predicting the future (1990).

McNerney wanted to enlarge the Blue Cross role beyond its traditional one of passing money from health care purchasers to hospitals. He wanted the Plans to use their health care dollars to reward improved service effectiveness and appropriateness. And he wanted Plans also to support prepaid group practices as an alternative way of discipline the system to improve its effectiveness. Also, by challenging the Blue Cross status quo he, in our terms, hoped to prevent the pathologies of ideology. He wanted to spur Blue Cross into prepaid group practice involvement in order to take "a social movement that was becoming bureaucratic and stale and captured by the wrong interests and shake it up" (McNerney, 1990, p. 2). This shaking up is, in our framework, policy as repositioning. McNerney used the next several years to systematically raise his Board's consciousness about prepaid group practice. Then, in 1970, he forced a vote on the issue. This happened, in "a semi-hostile environment" (McNerney, 1990).

Such a utopian challenge to the status quo involved organizational politics. Over the years the main political cleavage—ideology as pattern— among Blue Cross directors in the 1950s and 1960s was between big and small (in terms of enrollment) Plans (Brockway, 1990). In this context, many directors in the 1960s were wary of McNerney's interest in prepaid group practice because it, as did his push for a Blue Cross role in Medicare, aggravated their fears of BCA becoming too powerful. It reminded them of John Mannix's drive for a national format for Blue Cross (Brockway, 1990). McNerney' selection had been backed by a key half dozen large Plans. He had to win the acceptance of the smaller Plans and their directors. Brockway recalls that McNerney skillfully built up board support by visibly consulting with the directors, often by phone, on critical decisions before he acted. One of the board's progressive leaders recalls, most of the Plan directors were either against prepaid group practice, ignorant about it, or regarded it as a nuisance. Generally, they reflected the ideology of their local medical society.

One former association executive who joined the Blue Cross Association in the 1960s recalls the traditional 1960s Blue Cross ideology and Plan reaction to prepaid group practice alternatives:

> We believed very strongly in the fee-for-service system, complete freedom of choice, and that we should not be involved in quality of care because it is a personal decision between the patient and his physician. Along comes [an alternative which] does not believe in fee-for-service, has a restricted list of providers and has a strong emphasis on quality of care.... Some Plan presidents had great difficulty. They did not believe in the concept.... It created a lot of anxiety in Plans.... [The problem] was predominantly attitudinal in nature. Blue Cross and Blue Shield [success was based on] selling American values.

When McNerney did speak out on prepaid group practice it caused some outrage. "Many of the Plan directors, some with power, were disturbed and let McNerney know...it was a high risk thing" (Brockway, 1990). Also in the 1960s some Blue Cross Plans were under mounting criticism over hospital costs and plan management practices. In a 1964 court case, the judge expressed concerns over a Blue Cross rate setting "labyrinth" and criticized state regulators for indifference to "mistaken facts, ficticious charges and, ficticious employees or even ficticious patients" (quoted in Law, 1974, p. 15).

McNerney faced similar resistance within the BCA staff. James Veney, who directed BCA's R&D Division in the mid-1960 recalls the challenge presented by the staff's traditional perspective. It was evident to him that McNerney's vision "was in fairly substantial conflict a lot of the time with the old guard. They had a tradition of doing business on the basis of the notion that hospital costs got covered—and not on trying to better understand how the system in the future should be developed or in what direction it should go" (1990). This led to some obstructionism forcing McNerney to move on certain fronts slower than he wanted.

As McNerney faced the Blue Cross confederation of independent Plans in the 1960s, it lacked both a relevant language for constructive change and a change-embracing attitude. Therefore, he prepared the way for overt action by first changing the language and in so doing helped to change Blue Cross' attitude towards change. This was a period for getting ready for a pivotal move that would begin to reposition the Blues. I will use Kenneth Burke's "dramatistic hexad"—which Burke (1968) observes is similar to

Talcott Parson's action system elements—to help organize a review of McNerney's rhetoric as expressed in various reports to the Blue Cross Association Board, speeches and articles, as they developed in the 1960s leading up to his "radical" 1967 public call for a study to evaluate the advantages and disadvantages of the prepaid group practice format of health care delivery and finance. Burke succinctly presents his pentad: "For there to be an *act*, there must be an *agent*. Similarly, there must be a *scene* in which the agent acts. To act in a scene, the agent must employ some mean, or *agency*. And it can be called an act in the full sense of the term only if it involves a *purpose*" (Burke, 1968, p. 446). To this Burke adds "*attitude*," that he derives from Mead, the pragmatic sociologist. I will use "attitude" to refer to the six ideological and utopian outlooks of our template. McNerney tended to stress agent and scene. He tried to redefine both the role, (i.e., identity of Blue Cross) and the social situation with which it interacted.

1964

In 1964 McNerney gave a speech to health care management students and researchers at the University of Chicago on the role of Blue Cross in cost and quality control (McNerney, 1964).

Scene. The article called attention to "storms of discontent" (p. 49) over rising hospital utilization and costs, noting the pressure from organized labor and other critics on the health care system. It cited as an example, union demand that prepaid group practices be established in order that workers have a health benefit alternative option. It then argued that the present health care system had some merits and reflected America's economic and political makeup.

Purpose. The purpose was scene-generated. Blue Cross served the community and the public. The article called for a Blue Cross hospital relationship that provided "orderly growth and operation according to community need" (p. 49). The theme of community need evokes the CCMC report.

Agent. It asserted that Blue Cross would act in this turbulent scene with these purposes in mind. Blue Cross management must, it argued, know "the facts" about the health care system, its dynamics, and the effectiveness of various interventions on utilization. It viewed such knowledge as a competitive and political necessity. It would provide the base for "the quest for intellectual leadership." Key was that Blue Cross not be just a fiscal conduit, but play a "*control role*," (i.e., project itself into the health care field of social forces and reshape them). This reflects Selznick and Fuller's views on institution building as a creative process. It related that at a recent two-day workshop involving all Blue Cross plan presidents two things had become clear. First, that going back to the 1700s (i.e., to Franklin's founding of Pennsylvania Hospital) the government had been a partner in providing and financing health care; second that the need to play a control role was the first truly new task to emerge since Blue Cross was invented in the 1930s. So this control role—this reinventing Blue Cross—involved working with, being an ally to, government. Also, it argued, Blue Cross must play this role in the service of community-focused purpose. Here McNerney reinterpreted the past in order to find a tool useful in the present. "Voluntarism" in the future for McNerney would resemble what it had been in the Colonial past: a partnership with government, one in which voluntary organizations had to be more publically accountable.

Act. Blue Cross must, it stated, in alliance with government, "mold" utilization (p. 55) and lead intellectually in being accountable to constituents and in policy formulation. It called for action and experimentation. Also, as noted above, leaders had to get the facts.

Agency. It reported on various Blue Cross Plan initiatives: claims review, certification of need for hospitalization, education programs, utilization review committees and area-wide health planning. It did not include any mention of prepaid group practice activity.

Attitude. It urged that this situation be seen accurately and not in terms of "wishful thinking" or "tired prejudice" (p. 49). Thus, it advocated building on the healthy ideological aspects of health care voluntarism, while rejecting its distortions ("tired prejudices") and utopian magical, fanciful thinking. Interestingly, although McNerney saw the need for Blue Cross to be the agent of enhanced orderliness, he also argued for the preservation of some of the health system's "looseness," with "enough give and take for experiment and action" (p. 52). The uneasy health care equilibrium was becoming more tenuous—and Blue Cross was becoming more of an anxious organization. And Blue Cross had to come to terms with change. (Interestingly, in the 1960s Reuther tried to get Detroit to build an energy-efficient small car so that America not lose business to foreign alternatives. He had less success than McNerney's limited success of making a parallel health care innovation argument.)

1965

Next, McNerney (1965) published a *New England Journal of Medicine* article "The Future of Voluntary Prepayment for Health Services."

Scene. This article began by observing that America was going through an "era of redefinition" marked by swift change in most social spheres: education, work, human relations, urban living and the relationship between government and people's health. All these areas had become explicit public policy concerns. It next went on to note that health care redefinition focused on voluntary prepayment, under which he included not only Blue Cross and Blue Shield Plans, but also prepaid group practice plans. It cited the growing numbers of people covered by health care insurance—more than three quarters of the population—and concluded that coverage of the population was approaching the saturation point. It then identified a paradox: with this "impressive growth" came a "depressive anxiety." Medicare legislation was percolating in Washington; there had been five years of experimentation with controls such as utilization review; a better mesh between public and private sectors was needed; and the poor were not protected.

Purpose. Health had become a personal, institutional and moral purpose. Communities, it noted, viewed "...their health institutions with more than a little pride. They are seen as an integral part of the 'complete' community." And as most people get access to care, it starts to be seen less as a need and more as a right. In other words, the symbolic meaning of health care was changing.

Agent. Both government and voluntary institutions are expressions of democratic communities, that is, agents or tools. It then called for health care "spokesmen" who could transcend narrow self-interest. The question again was one of role. Prepayment should not, he argued, be seen as either government or private, but as some creative compromise or combination of the two. It saw this as requiring pragmatism and political art.

Agency. The article took an interesting stand on the issue of public/private roles. He observed that government from time to time will create or use an established intermediate organization to accomplish a public purpose by means of a private endeavor. It cited the American non-profit hospital as an example.

Act. It warned that health care is inherently costly. It called for negotiation over public policy and reforming what was performing weakly, while preserving what was working well. It identified area-wide planning and utilization review as specific things to encourage. Here it was placing his policy bias in repositioning health care skills to achieve some gains.

Attitude. It argued that there was no "magical solutions" but incremental changes that fit our particular pluralistic culture, that is, avoid the worst of utopian thinking. McNerney stressed that action should focus on the concrete problem of getting something done in the public interest.

1966

Scene. In a 1966 speech—"Comprehensive Personal Health Care Services: A Management Challenge to the Health Professions"—to the American Public Health Association's 1966 Annual Meeting, McNerney reacted to the recently released Report of the National Commission on Community Health Service. An interesting refocusing of the context is contained here. McNerney noted that aggregated health care costs had become so large that increases would henceforth have to be justified in competition with other community needs.

Purpose. In this context McNerney saw a new need to protect the health care field from unsuccessful competition with other community needs for scarce resources. And the need was to learn how to get the American health care job done more effectively.

Agent. Given this scene and purpose, he asserted that health care was "managerially underdeveloped." McNerney then took a general leadership theme from the National Commission report to sketch out a new hero to provide "intellectual leadership." Intellectual leadership resonates with Pettigrew's (1987) stress on leadership being a battle of ideas and ideologies. The spokesman of McNerney's 1965 article was to go beyond public relations and self-seeking. Now he gave this leader a name: *statesman.* Statespersons must, he suggested, understand the workings of the economic, political, as well as health care systems. Further, they would have to become masters of the administrative process as well as be adept at working the community power structure. Plus, the statesperson would have to understand individual and group behavior. In short, here is a Deweyan interdisciplinary actor. As McNerney urged in 1964—the health care leader as statesperson must "know the facts." This resonates with both the CCMC and Selznick's "statesman."

Agency. McNerney suggested that the nation needed a select group of graduate university programs in health administration to produce such statesman. They, in turn, would effectively "plan for people...make systems work for people." This appears top-down.

Act. McNerney called for experimentation.

Attitude. He pragmatically urged that the field did not have to wait for full philosophical certainty prior to action, but should act when there were opportunities to explore the possible.

1967

Scene. In his 1967 annual report to his board, McNerney (Blue Cross Association, 1967a) took note of the explosive growth in business resulting from the Medicare contract and labeled the time as an era of public policy negotiation. Cost and delivery were now subjects for public policy debate.

Purpose. Solutions to health care problems that fit the American culture had to be found. These solutions had to based, he reiterated, on information. He argued that the Blues should be honest enough to keep what was working and replace what did not work.

Agent. McNerney asserted that Blue Cross executives must do more than perform their traditional prepayment role and manage their growth. They had to also act as health care statespersons and get the facts about various organizational forms of rendering health services. The public, he argued, had a right to know about, for example, the advantages and disadvantages of prepaid group practice.

Act. He then called for objective studies of the effectiveness of various forms of medical practice.

Agency. And he called on the AMA and the AHA to do such studies.

Attitude. This annual report is interesting because McNerney carried ideas he had expressed externally back into the Blue Cross confederation, and he added the politically bold step of challenging the more powerful and established national health care trade associations to undertake the health services evaluation studies that were likely to upset the health care status quo. He was, then, using research fact-finding as a way to undo ideological distortion and to prod the field into preliminary action. This was a utopian challenge to established authority. As Pettigrew (1987) would say, McNerney had redefined and mobilized BCA's environment in order to pressure Blue Cross into constructive change. Again McNerney argued that there were no "magical solutions," but rather a need to "know the facts."

A Deweyan Connection: A North Star

I want to take a brief look at community service as a purpose. This was the consideration to which the progressive BCA search committee that chose McNerney owed their loyalty. "Community service" is a central theme in McNerney's writing and speeches. This is the moral value that he tried to reinfuse into the Blues' organizational character. McNerney observes, echoing Stuart (1953):

> It is very important to say that adaptation is the rule of survival in organisms, institutions, whatever. However, this does not imply that you react to the wrong forces or that you overreact. The important thing is to know where your North Star is and in my opinion for the Blues it was community welfare, of which the hospitals and doctors were a part, but not ends in themselves. Yes, Blue Cross had to be adaptive but never at the expense of a mission that dedicated itself to better community health. (1990)

This means that adaptations such as prepaid group practice, control role, cost containment, and so on, were all, to use Dewey's distinction, ends-in-view and never for McNerney ends-in-themselves.

McNerney's notion of "community" as a North Star is clarified by something Dewey wrote when he tried to illustrate what he meant by ends-in-view:

> A mariner does not sail towards the stars, but by noting the stars he is aided in conducting his present activity of sailing. A port or haven is his objective, but only in the sense of reaching it, not of taking possession of it. The harbor stands in his thought as a significant point at which his activity will need re-direction.... The port is truly the beginning of another mode of activity as it is the termination of the present one. (1964, pp. 72–73)

Using "community service" as his North Star, his basic consideration, McNerney was able at the beginning of the "management and control era" (Anderson, 1985) to see that the emerging move towards efficiency and economy were not ends-in-themselves, but simply the next harbor in the evolution of American health care. Arrival there would bring new problems and embarking towards further policy ports of call.

Mediating Between Ideology and Utopia (1967–1969)

In 1967 McNerney was awarded the American Hospital Association's Justin Ford Kimball Award in recognition for outstanding service to hospital prepayment. He was at the time just turning forty-two years of age. The time was one of social movements and upheaval, of a generation gap. McNerney made social change the theme of his acceptance remarks. He clearly sympathized with the young whom he saw as both idealistic and pragmatic. He wanted to see American society change without excessive strain. The Deweyan point is that he presented himself as a mediator of *ideological and utopian attitudes*: "Let us hope that the key decision-makers can borrow intelligently from the predictions and predilections of the young and old so that change is matched with stability, dash with wisdom and the need to create with the need for structure." Here McNerney was combining Rorem stability with Mannix swashbuckling.

In the late 1960s McNerney first exhorted in 1967 the AMA elder statesmen to consider change; that is, be less ideological and then two years later prodded prepaid group practice advocates to be less (youthfully) zealous, that is, be less utopian. Such social mediation is clearly not "pragmatic" in the sense of political expediency. It is "pragmatic" in Deweyan terms: critically exploring the present's possibilities in a quest for community. McNerney was operating as a health policy "gadfly" prodding all parties to explore possibilities.

In the mid-1960s, McNerney had come to terms with change. He had argued that health care statesmen as intellectual leaders needed to get and share the facts about prepaid group practice. Late in 1966 he tried to shift from adjusting attitudes to stimulating action about prepaid group practice. The question in our framework is how *do* you explore possibilities? How do you explore what is possible? Clearly organized medicine and many Blue Cross executives had felt for decades that prepaid group practice was "impossible"—and had the ideological power to enforce this feeling. This suppressed the possibility of innovation. The question becomes, then, how do you combat such an ideological self-fulfilling prophecy. McNerney's answer is that, in our terminology, a *utopian self-fulfilling prophecy may defeat an ideological one*. Recall McNerney's assertion "If you think about it, the self-fulfilling prophecy is a valid notion. You are what you think of yourself" (1984, p. 55).

Guy Benveniste (1989) has spelled out the dynamics of utopian self-fulfilling prophecies. The challenge of exploring the possible is to gain credibility for an innovative idea. The trick, he argues, is to build a "bandwagon" which creates a "multiplier effect," that is, "when an idea catches on, when support for a new course of action multiplies, when indecision evaporates and individuals or groups decide to move ahead in a given direction" (Benveniste 1989, p. 130). In short, the multiplier occurs when a shared belief in the inevitability of the course of action (or idea) is created. There is then a welling up from the bottom of support as people want to get on the bandwagon, that is, associate with a winner. Benveniste breaks the process into three elements: floating the idea, triggering the multiplier and the multiplier itself. Floating the idea involves letting it surface, creating awareness of it. Just saying the idea prods it closer to actualization. Discussing it is yet another step. Floating begins to create legitimacy for an idea. It is, Benveniste stresses, a step-by-step learning process. Triggering the multiplier is an event which involves three things: building a technical case for the concept, a visible coalition of supporters and a symbolic stance toward the idea—for example, "an idea whose time has come." The media will hopefully follow the floating of the idea and carry the message to potential allies. This adds further legitimacy to the idea.

In the late 1966, McNerney continued to build a prepaid group practice bandwagon. He had earlier in the 1960s publicly floated the idea by simply mentioning it and being willing to publicly discuss it. Now he moved another step. He publicly suggested that prepaid group practice should be studied—and the study should be funded by the federal government. Prepaid group practice was worthy of inquiry. McNerney instructed James Veney, Director of BCA's Research and Development Division to design a proposal for a research project that would seek to scientifically pin down whether prepaid group practice plans offering ambulatory care services had a causal relationship with the reported lower hospital admissions rates observed at these plans (McNerney, 1990; Veney, 1990). The proposal was finished by March of 1967. Its methodology was to compare the in- and out-patient utilization rates of two 1000-person samples drawn from the Federal Employees Benefits Program (FEP). One sample was federal employees enrolled with the D.C.-based prepaid group practice, Group Health Association. The study was to take three years (1968–1970) and cost nearly $300,000. BCA intended to use the proposal to seek funding from HEW's Public Health Service.

On March 7, 1967, Veney and Harold Pearce, BCA vice president, met with FEP officials to seek their support of the project. Joseph Harvey, the director of the Blue Cross Association-National Association of Blue Shield Plans (BCA-NABSP) FEP account, was invited to the meeting. Since the FEP national account was a joint BCA-NABSP activity, he reminded Veney and Pearce that the proposed study would involve Blue Shield data and interests. Therefore a week later Veney contacted Waldo Stevens, NABSP vice president, to describe the study and seek NABSP support— or at least have NABSP not oppose the project. Stevens registered his surprise that BCA had not involved Blue Shield earlier. He requested a copy of the proposal to review before taking any position on the study. On March 28th Veney gave Stevens a copy and invited him to join a meeting at the University of Chicago's National Opinion Research Center to discuss the project's methodology.

Several outside health care research experts were meeting participants. Stevens came away with a clear impression that the experts were all pro-prepaid group practice who hoped that the study results would be favorable to that alternative health care format. It was only at this meeting that Stevens learned about the earlier BCA contact with FEP. A week later he sent a memo to his boss, Executive Vice President John Castellucci, recounting these events and taking strong exception to BCA's taking unilateral action in an area of known mutual interest. Castellucci, on April 7th, wrote McNerney about the matter. He adopted Steven's reservations as his own and added: "I am certainly not opposed to studies that will produce information that will be helpful to both Blue Cross and Blue Shield. However, I think before any attempt is made to obtain a government grant which makes the results of this study public property...a more thorough discussion should be had with NABSP." Here was the issue: McNerney, the statesman, thought that the public had a right to the facts. Castellucci saw the facts only within his organization's interests. This was policy as prod versus pattern.

Let us look at this idea of a prepaid group practice research proposal. The idea had several political implications. First, it implied that a significant amount of hospitalization was wasteful (Stevens, 1989). This would be upsetting to the American Hospital Association which still controlled the Blue Cross logo. BCA had always been AHA's "stepchild" (Rorem, 1988), so the proposal was a way of declaring BCA's growing up, that is, becoming truly independent—attaining its own identity. The study also suggested that perhaps fee-for-service, solo practice had no monopoly on quality, affordable health care. So, it was bound to upset organized medicine, and consequently, Blue Shield. Looking further into the future, the prepaid group practice concept had two additional implications. First, it combined finance and delivery—which had been kept separate in twentieth-century American health care organization. Second, it provided a single point of accountability for medical and hospital care coverage— while the traditional Blue Cross Plan, Blue Shield Plan arrangement bifurcated accountability. Given all these politically sensitive points, suggestion of prepaid group practice inquiry was bound to lead to fierce political "discussion"—that is, it would shake things up. Inquiry was a prod to challenge the status quo.

McNerney, while directing the Michigan health services research project in the 1950s and the AHA-BCA study of the aged earlier in the 1960s, had learned that outside the normal methodological processes of studies there are "a lot of political eddies and currents" (1984, p. 122). He had learned that just because it seemed a good idea to research a topic that by no means guarantees that people will share your viewpoint and cooperate. Research requires political leadership to "pave the way" and deal with conflict created. McNerney recalls, "the prepaid group practice study was not only a political thing. My feelings were that it was a subject that could be discussed forever emotionally, but if we could get some facts, not speculations, on quality and usage, then this would considerably focus discussion and silence the false critics" (1990). The prepaid group practice research idea was an attempt to repeat his prior success with research in a volatile political environment. His idea was to get the facts, publish them and thereby enlighten public debate. While he shared the CCMC's faith in fact-finding, he brought to inquiry Franklin-like publicist skills in presenting the facts politically. McNerney felt that facts effectively communicated could neutralize the false critics' ideological distortions.

On April 27th (1967) McNerney held a press conference in Washington, D.C. where he went public with his views on group practice and prepaid group practice research. He refused to allow Blue Shield to slow him down at this point on prepaid group practice fact-finding. The BCA press release's headline read: "Blue Cross President Predicts Spread of Group Practice, Greater Controls and Planning to Curb Health Cost Rises" (Blue Cross Association, 1967b). Group practice, regionalization, prepaid group practice—these things are precisely what the Committee on the Costs of Medical Care had called for thirty-five years earlier. McNerney here was in effect calling for a reversal of Dr. Fishbein's ideologically labeling of these things as radical utopian fantasies. McNerney declared that they *were* possible and desirable. He was forecasting a workable future.

In his remarks and in the press release, McNerney focused on group practice and used *prepaid* group practice as just one illustration. Using an "innovative argument" (Stewart, Smith & Denton, 1984, p. 26), his rhetoric simply swept aside any notion that the innovations he proposed could not or would not work. He predicted that group practice would flourish. He continued: "Speculation on whether such ideas as group practice are usable is over" (Blue Cross Association, 1967b, p. 1). Now such an innovative argument often elicits charges that it is impractical, unwise or radical. Indeed, one of the reporters asked McNerney if he was predicting the end of fee-for-service medicine. McNerney was quick to deny this radical implication. He noted that while the demise of the traditional mode had been predicted since the 1930s (i.e., since the CCMC) it was still the dominant pattern. He did note, though, that group practice was "strong and vigorous." McNerney suggested that the country was "going, on a cyclical curve, to return to look harder at this concept of organization of medical practice."

Using an innovative argument McNerney put this reexamination in terms of a nagging discontent with the established order and a preference for change by experiment. He cited the continuing problems of health manpower shortages and costs. He further legitimated his prediction by citing President Johnson having HEW Secretary John Gardner call three national conferences of experts to tackle the problem from three angles: cost, group practice, and prepayment. McNerney also stressed what he called a "silent conspiracy in the public interest": young physicians were not finding solo practice satisfying and were beginning to talk about group practice. Here he was attacking the distorted view that all physicians supported the status quo. He reframed the issue as one of productivity. He suggested that the way to improve productivity was to seek new medical care organizational formats. McNerney noted that group practice had been traditionally "untouchable." He called on the AMA and AHA to sponsor research on group practice.

Looking at McNerney's notion of health care association leadership, we see him in this conference:

- acting as a *critical* force speaking out about healthcare costs;
- being an *educator* is addressing the public about possible remedies;
- being a *gadfly* in challenging the AMA and AHA to conduct research on prepaid group practice;
- *communicating* effectively in expressing complicated issues by means of metaphors such as "silent conspiracy";
- *framing* the issue as one of the need for improved productivity.

The final rhetorical irony found in this press conference is that McNerney, in effect, reversed Fishbein's conspiratorial argument. Fishbein had suggested that health care reform was an un-American conspiracy. McNerney asserted that it was a plot in the public interest. They both exaggerated the public support against and for their respective "conspiracies."

Early in May, HEW Secretary Gardner sent McNerney a supportive letter agreeing with the thoughts McNerney had expressed at the press conference. McNerney, the gadfly, responded, pledging to stimulate further public discussion of group practice and the need for greater health care efficiency. He assured Gardner of his determination "to commit our research facilities to studies of the effects on health care of various organizations of medical practice and benefit structures. Also, we are defining and extending our control mechanisms and benefits to promote more effective use of health services and facilities" (May 3, 1967). In late May, BCA submitted the prepaid group practice research proposal to HEW.

On June 1, Dr. Ackerman, National Association of Blue Shield Plans (NABSP) Board Chairman, sent board members a memo expressing his concerns over McNerney's press conference and its implications for Blue Shield. He attached a copy of McNerney's press release, a transcript of the questions and answers, a *Washington Post* (Auerbach, 1967) article on the conference, the letter from John Gardner, HEW Secretary, to McNerney, and McNerney's reply. Ackerman also quoted *Washington Post* coverage. On June 18, 1967, NABSP's Executive Committee reviewed BCA's request for participation in the study (or nonopposition) in the context of McNerney's recent press conference (National Association of Blue Shield Plans, 1967a). It decided to officially oppose the study. It took McNerney's group practice prediction as an endorsement of "closed panel practice as a suggested solution for reducing the cost of medical care." This contrasts with what McNerney had actually said. He predicted the growth of group practice per se, while mentioning prepaid group practice formats as simply one alternative. It is clear that *prepaid group prac-*

tice was an unmentionable. McNerney's making it a topic for discussion had shaken up the status quo. The AMA and NABSP would try to suppress the concept as a consideration in health policy discussion.

We have here echoes from the 1930s controversy over CCMC's recommendation of group practice and its prepaid variant. As organized medicine back then suggested that there was a need to look at more factors, NABSP here argued that the proposed study made cost the paramount factor and tended to ignore quality of care and public satisfaction. Like the AMA attack on the CCMC majority report, NABSP criticized the proposed study as being biased as indicated by McNerney's press conference statements. Also, much of organized medicine criticized the CCMC report in terms of alleged previous statements by some CCMC members, here too a document was interpreted not on its own terms, but in the context of vague readings of other external statements by its authors.

NABSP suggested that the publicity generated by the BCA press conference indicated a "preconceived bias and seems to represent an effort to influence public and official opinion before the proposed study is made." Also, NABSP noted that "the advanced statements on the study evoke a strange contrast between what the sponsors of the study may want and what the public has preferred to select over the past thirty years." But the public had been denied by organized medicine in most communities an alternative choice to the traditional fee-for-service format. NABSP was being ideological here in masking organized medicine's pattern of powerful activities to preserve the status quo. This was built into the existing pattern. Finally, the Blue Shield statement closed by taking exception to BCA's unilateral approach and voted to communicate its opposition to the study to both the BCA board and to all Blue Shield Plans (NABSP, June 18, 1967a).

Many NABSP Board members—physicians—stayed over in Atlantic City for the AMA's annual convention (June 18-22, 1967). McNerney and HEW's Wilbur Cohen, ran into severe criticism at the opening session of the AMA's policymaking House of Delegates (HOD). Resolutions made at this opening session were then sent for two days of discussion by reference committees with final votes taken by the 230 delegates on the last day of the convention. Resolutions included calls for the investigation and/or firing of HEW Secretary Wilbur Cohen for his push for national health insurance. In this heated atmosphere, the California delegation argued that BCA leadership had no business meddling in the private practice of medicine. They asserted that the AMA and the NABSP had not been informed in advance of the study proposal. They suggested that the BCA consider limiting its public statements to hospital care and not discuss medical care until it consulted with the medical profession. Similarly, they opposed the use of federal funds by BCA for medical care delivery research unless such studies involved AMA and NABSP representatives (Blue Cross Association, 1967g, p. 1). The House of Delegates adopted a resolution made by the delegation and forwarded a copy to the secretary of HEW.

On September 18, 1967 a letter from the office of the secretary of HEW to the AMA questioned the propriety of the House of Delegates request to deny HEW funding of the BCA proposal and rejected the House of Delegates' request. This was reported to the House of Delegates in November when it met in Houston. While the AMA Board accepted in general the need to study various health care delivery approaches, it urged the House of Delegates to again request that HEW and all people involved in the research grant proposal process reject the BCA proposal because it was sponsored by only one organization and McNerney's public statements were clearly biased.

On June 23, the BCA Board met. The proposed study of group practice was the fourth agenda item. Present were Castellucci and NABSP Board Chairman Dr. Carl Ackerman, M.D. The BCA Board then discussed the NABSP June 19th telegram that had communicated the NABSP position to BCA and all Blue Shield Plans. The BCA Board consensus was that "this study and other studies...should be undertaken from time to time" (BCA, 1967d, p. 3). The next month HEW Secretary Gardner's first national conference on medical care costs was held. Unlike 1932, the sky did not fall in after the AMA had opposed prepaid group practice. On July 25, Dr. Ackerman convened the NABSP Executive Committee to discuss, in light of BCA's going forward on the prepaid group research proposal, the need to redefine the relationship between the NABSP and BCA (NABSP, 1967b). A week later the media reviewed the issue. *Medical World News* (Blue Cross presses for study, August, 1967) presented events as a story of BCA being interested in fact-finding, while the AMA, a long-standing opponent of prepaid group practice, opposing the study. The article depicted the issue as naturally flowing out of a previous study done by the Federal Employees Benefits Program which contained statistics revealing an apparent difference in hospital utilization rates in employees under conventional Blue Cross coverage and those under pre-paid group practice plans. The obvious practical question posed by the statistics was "why?" Dr. James Veney, Ph.D., BCA's research director argued that as the nation's largest private health insurer, Blue Cross, had a natural need to answer this question. The *Medical World News* article then observed that "The very raising of such questions is unsettling to Blue Shield and to many proponents of solo practice" (p. 28). Veney went on to lament what he took as organized medicine's defensively emotional reaction to a straightforward attempt to "find out something."

A few days later the *National Observer* (Western, 1967, August 28) ran a front page story on prepaid group practice focusing on the confer-ences that HEW Secretary Gardner was convening "to *prod* the medi-cal profession to form new group practices. Government experts contend that this may be the best means of providing comprehensive, high quality care at the lowest possible cost" (p. 1, italics added). The article con-cluded by noting that reorganizing the American health care system along group practice lines might be the answer to rising health care costs. It added that a long test period would happen before such reform took place. In September a HEW conference focused on the potential role of health insurers in fostering the growth of group practice was held. The consensus at the conference was that insurers were now expected to help shape the delivery system into which they were pumping $10 billion a year. There was also recognition that there had to be research on vari-ous methods of health care delivery finance and delivery. The confer-ence called for insurers to participate in experiments and demonstrations. There was also a need for insurers to admit innovative alternatives into their offerings (*Blue Cross Association*, October 25, 1967g). This helped legitimize McNerney's press conference and prepaid group practice re-search proposal.

In late October, another HEW conference was held in Chicago. Here McNerney supported the ideas of public forums in which people at all levels could exchange views on group practice (*Blue Cross Association*, October 23, 1967f). McNerney sent all Blue Cross Plan directors copies of his own notes from the meeting. His cover memo (personal communi-cation) stressed the need to stop seeing prepaid group practice in charged terms of political extremes. He noted that "If the *conference accomplished anything, it was to make group practice a legitimate subject for conver-sation.*" (October 25, 1967, italics added).

The key point about this is that the ideological pattern of discourse that precluded discussion of "prepaid group practice" had been shattered. The *BCA Digest* item on the Conference also included the summarizing remarks of the conference director, Dr. John Cashman, M.D. (PHS) who noted that even five years earlier, a national conference on group practice would have been impossible. This was McNerney's point that group practice had always been excluded from polite health care conversation. The established *pattern* of American medical care discourse had excluded the term.

The AMA Board of Trustees (American Medical Association, 1967b) in November recommended that the House of Delegates reiterate its objections to BCA about the proposed prepaid group practice research proposal. While the AMA Board expressed its general approval of research on various methods of organizing and delivering health care, it urged the House of Delegates to request that all those involved in evaluating the BCA proposal think twice before funding such a study by "a single agency whose impartial attitude is in doubt" (p. 198). Subsequently, the Public Health Service rejected the BCA request for funds the following May (PHS rejects Blue Cross request, May 6, 1968). Ironically, that November, Dr. Dwight Wilbur, AMA president, agreed with McNerney's 1967 prediction that group practice was a growth industry (Blue Cross Association, 1968, November 1). So at least an element of the AMA had hopped, if reluctantly, aboard the group practice bandwagon. As Benveniste points out: "Conflict also reinforces the multiplier. If there has been consistent opposition and the opposition finally gives up, belief in the inevitability of the outcome is reinforced" (1989, p. 136). In 1970, former BCA health researcher, Donald Riedel, now at Yale, with McNerney's support did get a grant from the Nixon administration's National Center for Health Services Research. The federal funds went to BCA's Health Services Foundation which subcontracted with Yale. A preliminary federal report was published in 1975 (Riedel, Walden, et al.). The final report, in book form came out in 1984 (Riedel, Walden). Clearly, politics aside—there was a commitment to inquiry.

In 1968 Robert Levine published an article in *Public Interest*. This article "Rethinking Social Policy Strategy" reveals an easily overlooked continuity between the liberal Johnson administration and the conservative Nixon administration. Levine reviewed the troubled history of the "War on Poverty" and suggested that the problem was in "the kind of incentives one can offer people and institutions to carry out programs that are socially desirable" (p. 87). The market incentives dimension of his view was picked up by Dr. Paul Ellwood as he fashioned his HMO strategy (Falkson, 1980). Levine's idea of social incentives was filtered out. 1968 was also a year marked by election year protest movement excitement and quiet group practice advance. In Rochester the local business community and Blue Cross Plan were beginning to develop a prepaid group practice, Harvard was doing the same thing in Boston. And the *New York Times* (December 8, 1968) carried an article announcing that the Kaiser Foundation Health Plan would assume control of Cleveland's 33,000 member Community Health Care Foundation (a labor-sponsored prepaid group practice plan started in 1962). Kaiser was moving east of the Mississippi. Further, a prepaid group practice was scheduled to open in Columbia, MD by the end of 1969.

Also in 1968, *Inquiry* published an article (Hedinger) which argued that the Blues had begun with a social philosophy orientation but that market forces had pushed it into a new commercial insurer-like identity. It asked whether a community service-oriented Blue Cross could survive in a for profit marketplace.

1969 marked a political irony. Vietnam prevented a continuation of the Johnson Administration and its liberal advocacy of prepaid group practice. The war also stimulated Nixon's conservative interest in the same phenomenon. As Starr (1982) notes, the Nixon administration also came under siege because of Vietnam. Nixon's survival strategy, Starr suggests, was to recast liberal concepts into conservative policies, Levine's article was incorporated into this strategy. In July of 1969 Nixon held a press conference where he stated that the American health care system was in a crisis condition, on the verge of breakdown (Starr, 1982).

A lengthy article on the Harvard prepaid group practice was published in the September, 1969 issue of *Perspective*—the Blue Cross system's nationwide health care magazine. In the article the Boston Blue Cross President stated his conviction that Blue Cross' role in the Harvard project—it would market the program to its accounts—could help shelter Blue Cross subscribers from skyrocketing health care costs. Moreover, Art Carty, Blue Cross vice president and a prime mover of the Harvard experiment, stressed HMO developing as a learning experience, an initial repositioning of his organization (Sheffield, 1970, September, pp. 11-12). This article went on to emphasize the local medical care politics of starting a prepaid group practice which included a slow, open, deliberative process of community coalition-building.

Also, in 1969 McNerney joined the Group Health Association of America's board. This was the prepaid group practice field's national trade association. He was sending a clear symbolic message: that he, and therefore BCA, regarded prepaid group practice as something legitimate. That June he gave the keynote address at GHAA's annual meeting (McNerney, 1969). There he briefly reviewed the medical profession's "emotional, often vitriolic attack on the concept" (p. 14). He gave the Deweyan diagnosis that such attacks were a symptom of "the unthinking application of old remedies to new and different problems" (p. 15). He stressed the need for new thinking to address new social and economic realities. He was critical of professional self-deception or ignorance.

After calling for more research on health care organization—McNerney noted BCA's research proposal to HEW and the AMA's condemnation of it—he moved on to note the need for the "courage to implement what we already know." He said it was time for his member plans to work with community-sponsored prepaid group practice projects. Like Carty, he saw a need to give prepaid group practice experiments a fair trial. He discussed removal of state legal barriers to prepaid group practice incorporation and the need for labor and management to offer these new options under collective bargaining dual choices mechanisms. He was calling for utopian repositioning.

One key theme of this speech was attitude. He suggested that prepaid group practice would be best served not by either the medical profession's defensive ideological protection of the status quo (which ignores new realities), or capricious utopian support. What it needed was a "fair crack at the market" (p. 16). Here he was pursuing the *via media*—the middle way between the extremes of ideological preservation of vested interests and the utopian fancy that one innovation fits all situations. Rather he stressed the need, echoing the Committee on the Costs of Medical Care's pragmatic experimentalism and sensitivity to a variation of community settings, to adapt the idea to local circumstances. He closed his speech by dismissing opponents of improved health care productivity as "old fogies" (p. 21) who foolishly evaluated alternatives in terms of nostalgia instead of results.

Also in July, 1969, President Nixon asked McNerney to head up a national task force to review the Medicaid program (Anderson, 1985). Nixon subsequently asked McNerney to expand the Task Force's scope to include the entire American healthcare system. In a few short months the

McNerney Task Force recapitulated for Nixon the learning experience of the Kennedy-Johnson administrations. Where McNerney had headed up a national fact-finding study of one group's health care problems, the aged, to start the 1960s, here he was ending the decade looking at the problem of another group, the poor. Where the passage of Medicare and Medicaid swiftly led to looking at the entire health care system, so too Nixon quickly asked McNerney to widen the inquiry and look at the entire American health care system. As the Johnson Administration discovered the impressive accomplishments of the Kaiser program and the potential of pre-paid group practice, so too, the McNerney Task Force ended up in June, 1970 recommending the innovation now called "Health Maintenance Organizations." Where the 1960s began with *Harper's* (October, 1960) identifying a health care "crisis," now Nixon ended the decade with his discovery: a health care "crisis." But now the solution would be "clothed," to borrow a McNerneyism, in marketplace garb.

3

Action: Experimentation
and Critical Decision (1970s)

The early 1970s began with turmoil over the Vietnam War and the Watergate affair. The 1950s dream of benevolent pluralism, Robert Wiebe (1975) has written, plunged in the anxious late 1960s and expired in the 1970s. In this period of endless unrest some people hoped that social problems might just go away if they could be ignored for long enough. Meanwhile, along with social agitation came a wave of social reforms, somewhat analogous to those of the 1950s, that often relied on private mechanisms. Some argued that public ends did not need public means. In general in the 1970s, bureaucrats and marketers were to be society's problem solvers. For health care the evolving watchwords became: "competition, private markets, managerialism and massive federal regulation" (Stevens, 1991a, p. 166).

In 1970 there was much health care optimism about the potential of the HMO concept. This was wasted in the three years it took to pass the HMO Act of 1973 (Falkson, 1980). The same year as the HMO Act, the Middle East oil embargo occurred. This "oil shock" triggered economic stagnation. As the economy slowed, doubts arose about the possibility of actively making headway on social problems. In health care policy doubts arose about the efficacy of medical care and proposed national health insurance schemes (Starr, 1982). By the end of the 1970s, many were judging the Federal HMO Act of 1973 an apparent failure (Brown, 1983; Starr, 1982).

A sense of this historical "up and down" cycle of optimism and pessimism can be captured by examining the evolution of the term "medical-industrial complex." Its origins can be traced to President Eisenhower's farewell address in 1961. Ironically, after the dull prosperity of the private-sector oriented 1950s, Eisenhower warned against the "military-industrial complex" (cited in Nisbet, 1988, p. 25). The military and the industrial sectors had, Ike warned, become too tightly linked and, thereby, constituted a dangerously powerful interest group, energized by money—what Carlyle long ago termed a "cash nexus" (Nisbet, p. 85).

In 1967, Robb Burlage, a policy analyst for Health PAC, carried Eisenhower's caveat into health care. Burlage introduced the phrase "medical-industrial complex" (Salmon, 1990). The phrase was then adopted by *Fortune* in 1970. In the January issue, its editors declared that "American medicine, the pride of the nation for many years, stands now on the brink of chaos" (p. 79). They asserted that only sound businesslike management could save the day and bring costs under control. One article recommended the Kaiser-Permanente arrangement as the new way to manage health care. Another article highlighted high-tech health care as a profitable, growing market opportunity—what it called "the medical-industrial complex" (p. 90). The issue then closed with a third article discussing the potential profits in hospital ownership. Thus, *Fortune*'s analysis had a 1950s-type optimism. It adapted Eisenhower's phrase, but ignored his warning.

Nonetheless, social anxiety quickly appropriated *Fortune*'s phrase. In 1971 the Health Policy Advisory Center exposed the darker side of the medical-industrial complex. It warned against the hazards of profit-driven health care: "But there is no reason yet to trust that the rationalizations that the health industry brings to health services will look like rationalizations to the consumer. Judging from America's experience with the drug industry, the consumer can expect no mercy from the new Medical-Industrial complex" (Health Policy Advisory Center, pp. 122–23).

So began a twenty-year era of "ruthless managerialism" (Stevens, 1991a, p. 167). Midway through this period, Dr. Arnold Relman (1980), editor of the *New England Journal of Medicine* wrote a famous article warning against the ascendant "medical-industrial complex." The academic element of the American medical elite was here, unknowingly, forming an unlikely alliance with the Health PAC consumer advocates. Eleven years later, in 1991, Relman completed a kind of cycle. He came out advocating prepaid group practice as the best way to re-organize American health care. It had taken the *New England Journal of Medicine* sixty years to endorse the Committee on the Costs of Medical Care's implicit recommendation of this concept.

In 1971 BCA itself was investigated by the Subcommittee on Antitrust and Monopoly of the Senate Committee on the Judiciary. This inquiry revealed that the association's assertion of quality control over its independent members was largely mere public relations. Some plans were excessive in providing top management with percs and rejected the association's authority to intervene. One CEO stated: "We run our show. They don't.... They have no control. We are a separate legal entity, run the show our way" (Law, 1974, pp. 22–23).

Two Models of HMO Policy Analysis

McNerney's warnings from the 1960s that the Blue's would have to respond to increasing public criticism by exploring the possible were borne out. Politicians now had new expectations about Blue Cross. Its activity on the prepaid group practice front had to be understood now in this light. Starr (1982) suggests that the label "crisis" both described and constructed a social reality: crisis demands action. And there was still some optimism that the American health care problem had some solutions. McNerney responded to public discontent by advocating some promising ideas such as prepaid group practice. On a "CBS Reports" television special, "Health in America," he said: "We have more to do. Our performance, so far, is spotty...I think that we should throw our weight behind better organization of medical practice" (Schorr, 1970, p. 99).

Having floated the prepaid group practice concept nationally on CBS, McNerney next moved to get it formally accepted by his Blue Cross confederation of plans, that is, he had to trigger an HMO multiplier. His approach was an action-oriented pragmatic one. This is clear if we juxtapose it with Dr. Paul Ellwood's (1971) famous HMO policy analysis, which followed a rational decision-making logic. First, we will describe Ellwood's decision-focused policy rhetoric.

The policy logic of decisionism has these four steps:

1. Identify objectives.
2. Identify alternative courses of action for achieving objectives.
3. Predict and evaluate the possible consequences for each alternative.
4. Select the alternative that maximizes the attainment of objectives (Stone, 1988, p. 5).

Ellwood's (1971) HMO policy analysis follows this model (see Miller, 1990). Its goal was to deal with the crisis of out-of-control costs and pay more attention to keeping people healthy. It looked at two alternatives:

government regulation or the creation of a self-regulating health maintenance industry that would obey market principles. The regulatory approach would have the principal negative consequence, it asserted, of
spurring health care inflation leading to national health insurance, or perhaps even a national health service. On the other hand, the market approach would lead to reorganizing the system to economically reward
providers for keeping people healthy. Obeying market forces, costs would
be controlled and the health care industry would self-regulate. Ellwood
called for a Nixon administration decision to adopt the Health Maintenance market strategy and avoid socialism. Adding to its appearance of
rationality, the policy analysis listed six specific action steps to implement the strategy. In Mintzberg's typology, this analysis was policy as
plan: a set of steps that take you from A to B.

Now as Brown (1983) has documented, the HMO Act was widely
viewed in 1980 as a relative failure evaluated in terms of *policy as a utopian master plan*. In 1980 there were just 230 HMOs in the U.S. covering only a small fraction of the population. On the last page of his book
he makes the Deweyan point that the HMO policy has nonetheless helped
to mediate the social transformation of American health care from its old
mold into something new and still emerging. This, I suggest, is policy as
prod. To use Starr's (1982) terminology, while the HMO *program* had
modest accomplishments, its *strategic indirect consequences* had considerable significance.

Looking at the Ellwood policy analysis a bit closer we find what Stone
(1988) might describe as a strategically crafted rhetorical argument. Essentially, we have in this analysis a narrative story of control. She summarizes such stories: "The situation is bad. We have always believed that
the situation was out of our control, something we had to accept but
couldn't influence. Now, however, let me show you that in fact we can
control things" (p. 113). Ellwood's "analysis" offered the reader hope. It
redescribed the world in a way that made problems solvable with tools at
hand, business tools in this case.

Ellwood redescribed health care problems largely in terms of economic
incentives that prepared its audience for economic-industrial solutions.
Dr. Ellwood's utopia rested on complete confidence in the legitimacy of
the marketplace. By using synecdoche—a figure of speech wherein a part
represents the whole—Ellwood used the actual and successful Kaiser-
Permanente HMO to represent all future, possible HMOs. The audience's

capacity for critical thought was thereby suspended by the policy rhetorician's poetry (Stone, 1988).

Clearly, Dr. Ellwood had transported the reader to the world of fanciful utopia. This radical utopian vision powerfully captivated much of the U.S. health policy audience. It also had them consider market-oriented alternatives, and thereby to explore the possible. He clearly challenged the medical status quo. He urged a rebellion against the established order of illness-oriented physicians regulated by government. He instead urged that health-oriented organizations compete in the marketplace. So we have here a market-promoting policy wrapped up in the symbolism of public health and its concern for health. And in good radical utopian fashion, Ellwood's analysis assumed an easy and efficacious reversal of motivation: in the HMO utopia doctors will be rewarded for keeping people healthy and not merely reacting to illness.

Unfortunately, Ellwood's analysis suffered the utopian pathology of the magic of thought. He simply did not deal with the practical problems of HMO institution-building in hundreds of unique communities across America. He had, to borrow Schon's (1971) phrase, no intermediate theory of community. As Ellwood once remarked to a group of Blue Cross executives: "The one thing I do wrong in coming before a group like this is come on too strong, implying it is just going to happen" (Ellwood, 1970, p. 13). One seasoned HMO development consultant spoke for many HMO pragmatists when he resisted Ellwood's utopian magical spell. The consultant objected that HMOs and HMO development were being depicted as "neat and logical engines all based on and fueled by the magic power of dollar energy.... Money motivations are turned upside down—doctors no longer prosper from disease; rather, wellness becomes the wellspring of pecuniary gain. But wait a minute.... Are we really talking about the real world we know? Or is this the logic of Alice in Wonderland?" (van Steenwyk, 1975c). This pragmatist insisted that HMOs were going to be started around the nation but out of complex local socioeconomic and health care forces and needs. At the national level Ellwood also ignored the realities of power and politics. Ten years after the HMO Act he admitted this: "I used to feel that there were some *magic* buttons in Washington. If they could be found and pushed, the medical care system could be transformed" (quoted in Iglehart, 1983, italics added).

Ellwood was, then, intellectual midwife to U.S. Federal HMO policy, which opened the door to the corporatization of American health care

(Salmon, 1975). He took a new policy perspective that stressed how economic incentives shape behavior and applied it to the American health care scene. This returns us to the pathology of ideology and its cloaking of social problems. While Ellwood's HMO utopia made a real contribution in allowing us to explore the possible and challenge the *status quo*, it also reinforced elitism while undermining successful innovation implementation. His utopia was used by others as an ideological cloak to hide elitism and profiteering. The HMO policy opened the door for the "medical-industrial empire."

The Blue Cross Association adopted a pragmatic approach to HMO policy analysis. At McNerney's request, in February 1970, Brian Heller, on BCA's Research and Development Division staff, took stock of where the Blues stood on prepaid group practice involvement. While Heller gathered these data on prepaid group practice from Plans, he also discussed with them their interests and needs. Based on this, he (personal communication) suggested to Anthony Singsen, research vice president, three short-term objectives: a meeting of all interested Blue Cross plan people; a workshop on the concept at the upcoming April annual meeting of Plans; and a series of specific, educational programs on the concept.

Workshops and similar events at BCA had evolved as tactical tools for managing change. As such they were carefully choreographed. They were meant to communicate to the Blue Cross Plans the general state of the art on some concept. And they were meant to motivate the Plan CEOs to accept the concept in terms of policy and action. This was part of the "salesmanship" mentioned by Selznick (1983). Often workshops showcased pathbreaking Plan CEOs in order to establish them as exemplars worthy of imitation, to build a bandwagon of support. Often a document was presented as a point of departure. Speakers were carefully selected in terms of peer respect, geographic distribution, and so on. A basic message was identified to be delivered to the audience by the event. Also a copy of a draft policy statement by McNerney was sent out. The workshop was designed to demonstrate that the "invisible conspiracy in the public interest" of 1967 was becoming manifest.

The first speaker at the two-day workshop (Blue Cross Association, 1970b) (April, 1970) was the president of the Massachusetts Plan, Henry D. Jones who conveyed the big picture: American healthcare problems, reorganization of delivery in the context of NHI, and marketing concerns. Next came J. Douglas Coleman, president of the New York City Plan who identified the primary challenge facing all alternatives as "one of creative imagination: development of constructive responses to problematic [local] issues" (Blue Cross Association, 1970a, p. 6). Perceptively he reminded his peers that a Blue Cross nondecision to offer such choices would lead local customers to search for some other organization to satisfy their needs. He closed by identifying Blue Cross' distinctive competence. It combined "organizational imagination" with administrative competence.

The third speaker was Dave Stewart, executive director of the Rochester, N.Y. Blue Cross Plan, who argued that Blue Cross action in the present would help it receive a role in the future. He was trying to get his colleagues to remember their community mission, accept change, and reposition themselves. Next came Leo Suycott, executive director of the Wisconsin Plan. He emphasized the realities of the marketplace. His customers were demanding that Blue Cross experiment with new alternatives. The cleanup hitter in the line-up of speakers was James Brown of the Los Angeles Plan. He summarized the key pressure points for change mentioned by the first four speakers. Their basic message was that industry, labor, government, consumers, medical educators, and some physicians all sought the development of prepaid group practice programs. This is why Blue Cross Plans had to hop aboard the ADS bandwagon. Brown was saying that it was time for Blue Cross to explore the possible.

Whereas Ellwood's (1971) policy analysis stressed what Burke (1968) termed agency and purpose (i.e., means and ends), McNerney's policy assessment stressed questions concerning scene and agent. He stressed the *situation* that Blue Cross Plans were finding themselves in and their role, that is, *identity*, in responding to market forces. Further, he sought policy approval as a means to spur *action*. This is the pragmatic logic of action (March & Olson, 1989)—of moral character, Dewey and Selznick would say—with its three questions which lead to action:

1. What kind of situation is this?
2. Who am I?
3. How appropriate are different actions for me in this situation?
4. Do the most appropriate (March & Olson, p, 23).

McNerney's six-page, single-spaced, prepaid group practice policy proposal (McNerney, 1970) followed this appropriateness logic very closely. Its first page and a half discussed the situation: the growth of prepaid group practice and the environmental reasons for this growth. The next one and a half pages dealt with "reasons for Blue Cross involvement" which flow from who Blue Cross is, its identity and image. After spending one page on what prepaid group practice is, it then concluded with a page on appropriate actions. After the workshop, McNerney took the prepaid group practice issue to the BCA Board in the form of a proposed policy statement "Blue Cross and Group Practice Prepayment" (McNerney, 1970) written by him with the assistance of BCA staffer Faith Rafkind.

What Kind of Situation is This?

The first paragraph began in a *via media* fashion. "In response to various economic and professional pressures, group practice has grown slowly over the years, underachieving in the eyes of its ardent proponents and alarmingly persistent to those who viewed it as inimical to sound medical practice" (p. 1). This helped separate him from the ideological debate over group practice. It then noted that interest in group practice had accelerated in recent years. It especially stressed increasing interest and involvement in group practice by some physicians. Thus it called attention to a division in the house of medicine on the topic—something Dr. Fishbein had long before obscured. The united *pattern* of established medical authority was crumbling.

In the second paragraph it quickly moved on to note that Blue Cross interest had grown apace. Here McNerney observed that some Blue Cross plans were already in the process of hopping on the bandwagon: four had established relations with prepaid group practices and nineteen others were exploring or actively negotiating with prepaid group practices. (This would account for roughly 33 percent of all the Plans.) This paragraph used an implicit ladder metaphor of involvement: Plans first became interested in prepaid group practice; they next study it; then they negotiate; finally they achieve operational status. The force of this metaphor is that all Plans would move from rung to rung.

The paper next presented the reasons for accelerated interest and growth. Its first point reflected Blue Cross' character of being market-driven. It then pointed out that both the public and private sectors were demanding better productivity and predictability of cost and access. McNerney identified *organization* as the key means of responding to this demand. Many of these points were basically the same as those made by the CCMC in 1932. The main difference was that by 1970 government and big business as large purchasers of health insurance were *beginning* to demand improvements in health care delivery and finance, The prepaid group practice bandwagon now had—at least *potentially*—an engine to pull it: the market.

The paper next argued for Blue Cross involvement. Here it gave reasons to move beyond floating the idea to trigger the multiplier with Blue Cross. He began with a call to action. "Now is the time for the Blue Cross Association to formulate an expression of policy and to assist Plans in implementation; in effect to give what has been a slow, disjointed movement greater focus and effectiveness" (1970, p. 2). McNerney then both predicted the future and artfully reviewed the present: "The forces described above are strong and varied: economic and social, as well as professional. They will intensify. Critically they are legitimate" (p. 2).

"Who" is Blue Cross?

The proposal offered a concept that linked the traditional Blue Cross way of life with the innovative prepaid group practice concept: "dual choice." ("Dual choice" is when the employer gives employees an alternative to the traditional health insurance plan offered as a fringe benefit.) He traced the growth of this concept since World War II. It thereby connected the innovation to the history of Blue Cross and its stake in national accounts. It next cited Ann Somers' argument that the dual choice mechanism was a force for innovation. It also mentioned the HEW Medicaid Task Force—McNerney was reminding his audience that he was directing it for the president at the moment—was thinking along similar lines.

With this mention of HEW the paper directed its audience's attention to the National Health Insurance issue swirling about the Blues. It warned: "If Blue Cross is to avoid the image, if not the fact, of limiting innovation inspired by consumers, it must support the concept and have available an alternative attractive to what is becoming a significant constituency" (1970, p. 2). It next showed that several prepaid group practice principles—service benefits, first-dollar payment, comprehensive benefits and community rating, were consistent with Blue Cross' historic objectives. In terms of our framework they were consistent with Blue Cross ideology's identity. It then reminded his audience that it was precisely these community-oriented principles that were "centrally related to Blue Cross' nonprofit standing before legislative and regulatory bodies" (p. 3). This was policy as perspective and pattern.

McNerney then made an essential triggering point: the "pressure for change is coming from the bottom up" (1970, p. 3). Here he intimated that there were allies out there ready to challenge the status quo. The paper noted that within the medical profession national groups were beginning to talk about the topic with more balance and a bit of cautious support. At the local level, he observed, many groups were "responding to their markets pragmatically within the context of definable consumer and professional problems.... The format discourages the old emotional debates which confused ethics with money and quality with quantity" (1970, p. 3). It was here arguing against ideologies that distort our perception of current problems (i.e., ploy) and merely preserve only self-interest (i.e., pattern). McNerney was trying to help local Blue Cross plan presidents view their own communities with the same pragmatic *via media* perspective as McNerney used in his opening sentences.

McNerney then connected this growth of pragmatic interest in prepaid group practice with federal legislative initiatives in health care finance and delivery system experimentation. He predicted that these would grow in priority and funding. He closed the section by stressing that the bandwagon was already in motion. He declared: "Experimentation has begun" (1970, p. 4). He argued that Blue Cross had to experiment or risk being left behind.

Appropriate Actions

The proposal then discussed group practice in a prepayment context and called again for evaluating its many variations. Then it discussed possible Blue Cross Plan roles in prepaid group practice ventures. It cited Plan experience to date and noted the pragmatic implementation principle of imaginative adaptation of concept to locale: "Blue Cross' role in concert with various group practice schemes varies with individual circumstances. Blues should flexibly use their organizational imagination to design alternative programs to fit local situations."

Finally, it presented a proposed policy position:

In contemplating a policy position, Blue Cross might consider reference to a few fundamentals, i.e.:

- No single delivery system will suffice for a nation as diverse as ours in terms of efficiency or as an answer to the many values being weighed by providers and consumers of care.
- In pursuit of greater efficiency and effectiveness of delivery of care and its financing, it is important that the consumer have available reasonable options so that his experiences can be a vital element in change.
- A health care system impeded by artificial restraints on experimentation or sufficient variation in implementation will ossify, in the end, resulting in problems of both cost and access.
- One worthy pattern of delivery of care is group practice, subject to various structures and methods of payment.
- Blue Cross should include such a pattern in its marketing plans and urge Blue Shield to consider the formulation of such an alternate benefit. (McNerney, 1970)

The first fundamental above raises the American value of pluralism. Our nation is diverse; answers to community problems various. The second is about the principle of liberty, freedom of choice in the market. This is a kind of "voting with your feet." The third principle implicitly attacks ideological dogmatism that hinders inquiry and thereby frustrates evolution and flexibility, leading to waste. The fourth identifies group practice, which he labels, a "worthy" approach, subject to many variations. The final point is that Blue Cross should include group practice in its offerings and urge its sidekick, Blue Shield, to do likewise. Notice that McNerney in this policy avoids the use of the term "prepaid group practice." As McNerney recalls: "I had to word that carefully. I wasn't saying that we should endorse prepaid group practice *per se*, but as a legitimate option in the marketplace." As he recalls, he won the board by just six votes out of almost 2000 weighted votes (McNerney, 1990, p. 2).

The BCA Board vigorously debated the proposed policy position (Blue Cross Association, 1970c). One group of Plan CEOs strongly argued that prepaid group practice was not a proper concern of Blue Cross. They held that Blue Cross should only offer established options. This echoes the AMA line from 1967 concerning Blue Cross prepaid group practice research. The other side accepted the need for experimentation: Blue Cross had a social responsibility to explore alternatives. They pointed out that some groups had withdrawn their opposition to group practice. They also stressed that group practice was not a monolithic thing, but consisted of a variety of formats. McNerney, from his travels, pointed out that across the country Blue Cross was criticized for concentrating too heavily on hospital coverage which had thereby de-emphasized ambulatory care services. He pointed out that Blue Cross' implicit position not to influence health care delivery (a nondecision) had had the effect of maintaining the established distorted delivery system. Its nonpolicy was, in our framework, policy as pattern.

The board passed the policy statement with an editorial change. In the fourth principle, the word "worthy" was deleted and "group practice" was qualified by the phrase "so-called." In short, "prepaid group practice" was not mentioned and reference to "group practice" was muted. Dave Stewart recalls the board discussion and vote: "McNerney won board 'support.' ...It was grudging acceptance or derogatory reaction. For those who voted favorably, it was something good for the other guy. If a Plan had no HMO competition, then it felt no pressure. Even some McNerney supporters on the board didn't get involved in prepaid group practice. Big business wasn't demanding it. And doctors were saying it was a bad idea" (Stewart, 1990, p. 3).

The rhetorical "trick" in this policy was in the word "option." A BCA executive at the time pointed out that McNerney as a health policy statesperson intellectually saw the need for an organizational alternative to discipline the dominant fee-for-service solo practice system, but as BCA President and Chairman of its board, he accepted working within the framework of a loose confederation of slow-to-change Plan presidents. Therefore, he translated "organizational alternative" into their operational-business perspective: prepaid group practices were "options," that is, products their customers were going to increasingly demand and get from some organization. So the Blue Cross CEOs "accepted" the innovation as merely another product line. Beneath this was, however, "the hidden metaphor" (Schon, 1979) of institution building that envisioned prepaid group practice as a tool to discipline and reshape American health care. Indeed, the subtext of the deletion of the word "worthy" can be interpreted as a way to deny this creative metaphor and the logic of action. As pragmatist Lon Fuller once asked: "Does this institution, in a context of other institutions, create a pattern of living that is satisfying and worthy of man's capacities?" (1981, p. 55). The board's equivocal action on prepaid group practice was a "critical decision" (Selznick, 1983, pp, 35–37) that is, one that would have long-term consequences for Blue Cross' organizational character and identity (Selznick, 1983; 1992). In the 1980s most Blue Cross Plans continued to react against this question about social worth.

McNerney was, as Gene Sibery (BCA's executive senior vice president and later Iowa Blue Cross president) recalls, leading Plan leaders where they didn't want to go (Sibery, 1988, p. 35). Shortly after the board approved the policy, McNerney called a meeting of all BCA professional staff. He told them that BCA was dedicated to the new HMO concept. He said it was the wave of the future. Anyone who saw it differently was, he suggested, free to seek employment elsewhere.

In his 1970 Annual Report (Blue Cross Association, 1970a) he stressed the growing consumer demands for health care reform (e.g., the American Public Health Association's Citizen Board of Inquiry) and mounting criticism of Blue Cross as self-serving in the press. He cited Jack Anderson's nationwide political column which commented: "Look at the cheek-to-jowl love affair between Blue Cross and hospitals." Also, he quoted New Jersey Governor Richard Hughes: "Blue Cross doesn't respond to the public.... It's controlled by large private hospitals." McNerney acknowledged that the American health care system had become self-serving. He called for a bold counter-move. And he argued for the Blues to stop defending the status quo and become reshapers of the health care system.

Later that month (May 26th) he sent his Board and all other Plan Chief Executives a memo following up on their approval of the policy statement in April: "At the Annual Meeting of Member Plans, April 1–2, 1970, Blue Cross and Group Practice Prepayment was a major topic on the program. On April 3, 1970, the Board of Governors approved a policy position which, *in effect, supported prepaid group practice as an alternative benefit*, subject to consumer option, and pointed to the need for *implementation* through product development and marketing" (italics added). Notice that McNerney here now trumpeted what the board had tried to mute: it was endorsing prepaid group practice as a legitimate option. Also note that he aggressively interpreted the policy as a call for immediate *action*. He then outlined upcoming educational events to implement the new policy, including an ADS Conference for June 9, 1970, to be held in Chicago. He also called attention to the possible need to adjust the Association's ADS policy to reflect the new federal HMO initiative.

The National Meeting on Alternative Forms of Health Care Delivery and Financing was jointly sponsored by BCA and NABSP (Blue Cross Association, 1970d). It had a very large turnout. Over forty states were represented. Attendees included a dozen chief plan executives. This paralleled the mounting excitement within HEW as the HMO policy bandwagon gathered steam there (Strumpf, 1990). McNerney opened the meeting by reiterating the points he had made at the annual meeting. He also mentioned emerging discussions and alliances with GHAA and the American Association of Medical Clinics—all around the prepaid group practice concept. He stressed the value of recent Blue Cross Plan experience in prepaid group practice plan development. He reviewed the Board-approved policy—reverting to his original wording which called prepaid group practice a *worthy* thing.

McNerney, in short, spoke on where Blue Cross was, where it wanted to go and how to get there. Strikingly, McNerney warned against HMO policy as ploy: "We should all be very clear that if variation is ever stretched to put some old ideas under a respectable cover...then we will have trouble, and we must guard against the possibilities assiduously" (Blue Cross Association, 1970d, p. 6). He closed by noting that "in Blue Cross' future, the delivery of services is our key, as it was when we started" (p. 7). Here he was arguing that prepaid group practice innovating was consistent with tradition. Here he was trying to take home to the Plans the present meaning of their past in order to turn them towards future institution building. He acknowledged that for many Plans this would involve a shift in perspective, plus the recruitment of new staff who understood how to set up ADSs. He closed with the announcement that the HEW had finally funded the prepaid group practice research study and that it would begin July 1, 1970. In September 23, 1970, the Kentucky Plan President, J.E. McConnel, sent a letter to McNerney, protesting McNerney's publicly stating that Blue Cross had endorsed group practice. McConnel wrote: "I think that, in view of the unrest in many local plan areas and the tightrope that many of us have to walk to be able to not only hold our position but to move forward, great care must be exercised to make sure your statements and those of your staff are reflecting individual views and not be mistaken to be that of the Board of Governors or of all the Plans" (personal communication).

In November the third phase of the educational process was held: a three-day meeting on ADS in Kansas City, Missouri (Nov. 17–19, 1970). This meeting took a workshop approach in which seasoned prepaid group practice professionals discussed specific technical aspects of PGP planning and operations (Blue Cross Association, 1970e).

The first speaker, Nathan Stark, stressed what he called "the climate—political, social and economic" (BCA 1970e, p. 3). He gave local medical society opposition or facilitation as a key political determinant. He stressed that program "organizers" needed to be able to bring together medical manpower, adequate money and competent managerial talent. He also addressed technical marketing and actuarial considerations. He reviewed the *slow* twenty-year climb to success of the Kaiser-Permanente program in Portland, Oregon. Next, GHAA's Louis Segadelli described how in the late 1960s GHAA developed an idea that the Public Health Service gave a small support grant. In 1967 with the PHS grant, GHAA placed a community organizer in Providence Rhode Island. Over the next few years the PHS increased the grant and thirty-three cities were on the GHAA list. Next David Neugent spoke about his Blue Cross Plan's dedication to being the health care leader in Wisconsin. The Plan was mindful of Federal interest in the HMO concept. He noted that Milwaukee was targeted by an HEW grant. He admitted: "We frankly saw some handwriting on the wall" (p. 16).

In the closing question and answer session, the first question—one that would haunt the Blue Cross HMO movement throughout the 1970s— was "Why should Blue Cross and Blue Shield go into competition with themselves?" (BCA, 1970e, p. 29). One Blue Cross executive's answer was direct and final: "I think it's a case of either losing existing membership or as a result of getting into group practice, keeping membership" (p. 29). Another Blue Cross panelist argued that Plan consumers wanted the option; the Plan should provide it. Another panelist suggested that the Blues consider an analogy to General Motors' strategy of offering several makes of cars (e.g., Chevy and Pontiac) that compete with each other. G.M. had thereby a variety of product lines to respond to different market segments.

In late 1970 a NABSP staffer reflected in a memo on the past year, his own reactions and those of Plan executives with whom he had talked: "The Plans seem to view prepaid group practice as essentially a marketing 'gimmick.' In other words, their interest in prepaid group practice essentially stems from its use as a dual choice option along with a standard Blue Shield contract option. My own personal opinion is that at this point in time we should not be concerned about Plan motivations in entering into prepaid group practice, but be more than happy that they want to get involved and support and encourage such involvement." This staff person noted that interested plans were seeking national association or consulting firm technical assistance. He shrewdly noted that BCA had gripped the prepaid group practice ball and had been leading for the past year by offering educational services. He suggested that technical assistance was the next leadership activity.

Blue Cross HMO Anxiety, Activity, and Action (1971–73): Policy Prods to Trigger an HMO Bandwagon

In February (1971) McNerney went public with his pressure on his own constituents. In *Forbes* an interview with McNerney ran under the telling title "Here's a president who criticizes his own outfit and wants the government to help him change it." Here McNerney revealed his statesman-gadfly self-image, identifying himself with the public: "The public is fed up with rising costs—and rightfully so" (p. 48). He asserted that BCA had hired him precisely because he was an "outspoken crusader" for health care reform. Briefly mentioning AMA resistance to reform, he also acknowledged that his own Plans' board members were mostly representative of providers and not of the general public. The article suggests that McNerney had to contend with resistance from his own constituency of Blue Cross Plans. "What we need," said McNerney, "is a top down crunch force. A question we've got to confront is whether the White House is going to help." He urged federal legislation to force action (*Here's a President*, p. 48).

In McNerney's 1971 Annual Report to his plans he described the public forces bearing down on the Blues to become more than a conduit of money to hospitals. National health insurance emerged as a top political issue: "It is highly likely that by 1972 or 1973 a bill will be passed... involving significant changes in the financing and delivery of health services.... We hear the question...are we more than a pipeline for provider money and aspirations? In some cases, we are not. In others we are too little more" (BCA, 1971a).

The clear implication was that Blue Cross had to do a new kind of job if it wanted to avoid becoming, to use Selznick's term (1983, p. 18) "expendable." McNerney's message was clear: Blue Cross would be held accountable to the public. They had, to borrow Selznick's (1983) words, to "symbolize the community's aspirations, its sense of identity" (p. 19). It is interesting to note McNerney's focus on language, his insistence that the word "accountability" became part of the Blues' basic vocabulary. He also realizes that this word clashed with a powerful traditional symbol of community identity: the hospital and its perceived self-interest. He argued here that the hospital become a "platform of voluntary leadership in health rather than a temple to acute care" (BCA, 1971a, p. 14).

With respect to Blue Cross' Plan ADS activity, the annual report noted that in the past year twenty-four Plans had been involved in ADS projects, six of which were operational. This was progress over the previous year's sixteen and four respectively. It noted six false arguments used by foot-dragging Plans: (1) ADS were only for poor people; (2) ADS development cost too much; (3) twenty plans cited feared medical community opposition; (4) Blue Shield hesitancy; (5) legal constraints; and (6) fear of repercussions from other groups such as labor. He swept these aside as mere excuses. The report asserted that the overriding obstacle was a lack of commitment by senior management who were simply not allocating manpower or money. It challenged them to break the inertia of their "wait and see" attitude (p. 15).

The annual report then, hit at Plan pride by noting that the world, including the Federal government, was "beating a path to Permanente's door." Kaiser, then, was the leader here, not Blue Cross. It touched a competitive nerve in his audience: commercial insurers were investing in prepaid group practice development. It then appealed to Blue Cross tradition, arguing that when Blue Cross founding fathers faced a similar situation in the Depression they set up their "own guidelines and plunged ahead. They did not wait for others to act" (p. 16).

The final argument focused on staying indispensable. The report suggested that the health care field's distinction between finance and delivery was "blurring." In such a changing situation, ADS would give Blue Cross some vital experience and expertise. This is precisely what Selznick (1983) had suggested. For an organization to maintain itself, to stay indispensable, it has to struggle to maintain its unique identity in facing up to new problems and altered circumstances. For Blue Cross this meant that it could no longer afford to be, or appear to be, co-opted (dominated) by the character of the hospital's interests and aspirations. Rather, it had to negotiate its accommodation with hospitals in light of community aspirations. To do this it had to develop new skills to take on its new ADS role. By building ADSs that reduced needless hospitalization, it was symbolically both serving the public interest and not serving mere hospital self-interest. But to be indispensable, it had to become *competent* as to ADS institution building. Moreover, in the health care future he projected, finance and delivery would be merged. Therefore, Blue Cross would have to acquire the skills to play a control role.

On August 12, 1971, BCA reluctantly passed its policy on HMOs (BCA, 1971b). This was sought by Association leadership in order to budget resources to staff and implement ADS activities at the Association. They had to play a careful political game in proposing the ADS budget (Sibery, 1990). The budget level was only as high as Association leadership thought the Board would tolerate. This policy supported HMOs as a promising ADS in the same spirit as the board's previous policy on prepaid group practice. It stressed the need for HMO planning to provide for consumer involvement, access to market, and overall local health planning considerations. The statement closed with three cautions. First, "There is no magic in HMOs." For cost and access problems to be tackled, real HMOs would have to be effectively organized, managed, and marketed. Second, HMOs in the foreseeable future would only provide a smaller portion of American health care. Third, the statement warned that HMO effectiveness would be dedicated to actually changing the delivery system and not just present the traditional pattern in some new guises. It warned, then, against policy as ploy or master plan.

The specter of NHI and Blue Cross' need for statesmen-salesmen to demonstrate the Blue's indispensability is shown in BCA testimony on HMOs presented to Senator Edward Kennedy's Senate Subcommittee on Health on November 2, 1971. Midway through the question and answer period after BCA Senior Vice President Eugene Sibery's presentation of BCA's HMO activities, accomplishments and policy, Senator Kennedy injected the issue of NHI. And he did so from an interesting angle. He charged that BCA was using subscriber funds to lobby in Congress. He asked Sibery about a confidential McNerney memo (September 10, 1971) sent to chief plan executives that described the need for a communications strategy to get the Blue Cross message across in light of emerging Congressional pressure for NHI.

> *Mr. Sibery*: We do not view this as a lobbying activity. It is a two-way communications vehicle. We feel there is considerable misunderstanding on the part of many people as to what Blue Cross is and what it has done...
>
> I think we are supporting some form of national health insurance...Blue Cross is a community institution, and will last only as long as it is useful to the community. If it should have outlived its usefulness then this would be understood. However, we honestly believe in our best judgment that it has a major continuing contribution to make and that its resourcefulness should be built upon in future activities. (BCA, 1971c)

Sibery here was defining an organization's right to sell itself, to show its "distinctive capability to produce a certain product or perform a special service" (Selznick, 1983, p. 139). As Sibery's remarks make clear, if BCA could not make this case, it would cease to exist. (Sibery also supported the idea that HMO boards be representative of their communities.)

In the media the association's ADS bandwagon got some attention. *Medical Economics* (a nationally circulated magazine for physicians) ran a story on the Blue Cross HMO bandwagon. It pointed out that while the federal government was still working out an HMO law, the Blues had about forty prepaid group practice projects in the works around the nation. It noted that some physicians were starting to approach Blue Cross Plans for help in launching their own projects. Given Blue Cross involvement, and sizable commercial insurance company start-up funding, the article closed by predicting "it won't be long before doctors in many more towns will see the bandwagon roll in" (Rosenberg, 1971, p. 267).

On March 6, BCA's Research and Development newsletter (circulated to all Blue Cross Plan CEOs and R&D departments) carried word that HEW had announced the first round of HMO planning and development grants. Funded projects were spread all around the nation. It also noted that fifty-one prospects had been funded in 1971. The message to Plans was that the federal HMO bandwagon was on its way to their locales.

On May 10, McNerney presented a BCA statement on HMOs to the House's subcommittee on Public Health and Environment (BCA, 1972b). Also testifying for the Blue Cross Plans were Rochester (New York) Plan President David Stewart and Wisconsin Plan President Leo Suycott. McNerney recited Blue Cross' past involvement with prepaid group practice and cited its 1971 policy statement on HMOs. Next he summarized the status of current involvement: ten Blue Cross Plans with sixteen operating programs, and thirty-eight at some stage of HMO consideration or actual development. He reviewed BCA recent educational conferences on HMO operations. He also stressed the idea that the dual choice mechanism was a grass roots pressure for health care innovation.

Next, McNerney offered an interesting set of practical observations and caveats in constructing HMO legislation including remembering "how complex and variegated this country and its health system are. Consumer attitudes and preferences vary widely as do the structure and traditions of the delivery system" (BCA, 1972b, p. 4–5). He stressed that HMO building would be difficult and time consuming. He went on to point out that

HMO policy objectives contained contradictions. HMOs were to increase comprehensiveness of coverage, but also reduced cost; they were to be more regulated to assure quality, yet they were expected to be innovative; sponsors of legislation wanted fast implementation while providing minimal start-up funding. He urged an action-oriented, social learning approach to HMOs. Although he approved of current policy discussion, he also warned against too much analysis: "We should make some judgments and take some risks, based on the public interest and what promises to work, and start, And, make changes as we go along, based on experience rather than endless speculation. Uncertainty should not lead to hesitation because potential gains outweigh the risks" (BCA, 1972b). Given limited available capital, McNerney suggested the pragmatic tactic of making maximum use of existing resources. He further called for the ingenious adaptation of general HMO models to fit varied local circumstances. He also warned against overselling the HMO concept.

After McNerney's statement, Stewart and Suycott made presentations about the practical aspects of their Plans' experience in HMO development. Congressman Rogers then asked the three Blue Cross people a set of questions. Two interesting points came out. First, the Blue Cross people stressed, in contrast to the Ellwood thrust, that HMO development required more than money—it required skills and organization. McNerney suggested that by using insurance companies as HMO developers the country could save waiting a five-to-ten-year-long period for university programs to generate an adequate skill pool.

The second point was that after the preceding five years of floating the prepaid group practice idea, physicians in general in various communities had become willing to let a handful of their colleagues get involved with small prepaid group practice projects, that is, let it be tried out in the local markets. Thus, there had been a shift from total resistance to an attitude of "O.K.—these ten guys can give it a shot." So, forty years after the Committee on the Costs of Medical Care recommendations—the medical community was ready to let the experiment begin.

Paralleling McNerney's HMO cautions were some warnings contained in Robert Levine's book *Public Planning: Failure and Redirection* (1972). This book was an amplification of his 1968 *Public Interest* article which had crystallized Ellwood's conceptualization of his HMO strategy (Falkson, 1980). In the book Levine argued that the 1960s Urban Renewal Program had had a decentralized marketing strategy. (This is precisely what the Ellwood-Nixon HMO strategy was: a market approach to re-structure a field.) But Levine in 1972, went on to suggest that it was Ur-ban Renewal's market strategy that was the source of its problems: "It uses the instrumentalities of and shibboleths of decentralization and pri-vate enterprise and uses them badly. Because the instrumentalities are powerful ones, their misdirection leads to powerful mistakes" (Levine, 1972, pp. 85–86).

Levine stressed the hazards posed by local self-seeking forces in imple-menting a marketplace strategy. The problem is, he suggested, that mar-ket strategies give inadequate consideration of local realities. He noted that market-oriented strategies do not effectively serve equity goals. And he suggested that these strategies can have unplanned (desireable or undesireable) consequences. Levine noted the interest shown in market approaches to health care reform as reorganization. He cautioned that this approach would "restore the pre-Medicare/Medicaid order in which the wealthy stood first in line and all others took what remained.... [It] should be recognized that efficiency has been substituted for equitable distribu-tion as the criterion" (p. 170). Levine here anticipated the access crisis of the 1980s. The danger of market-oriented strategies is that they encour-age us to skip over the recalcitrant local political-socioeconomic forces at work in real communities coast to coast. Levine's warning is against the dangers of utopian escapist thinking and ideological distortion, of hid-ing issues of implementation and self-interest.

Elwood's strategy was selectively conceptualized in terms generated from the War on Poverty experience. He and the Nixon administration dropped out the nuisances and cautions of the OEO policy analysts. Levine (1972) also suggested that social policies are packaged in terms of uto-pian myths in order to gain support. In this light the HMO strategy used the myth of the marketplace to deflect attention from the fact that the HMO strategy was going to be difficult to implement.

Levine pointed out a basic social justice problem posed in marketplace strategies: they shift the ethical criterion from equitable distribution of resources to the efficient allocation of resources. He demanded that we be honest about this and its consequences. In the recent twenty-year mar-ketplace turn of American health care policy, procompetition proponents were not honest about the social justice implications of market-oriented strategies and their stress on competitive advantage and profit maximi-zation. Inevitably market justice had the consequence of under-care and under-coverage in terms of health insurance. The final point to be made here is that Levine's book and McNerney's testimony offered the policy-makers and politicians pragmatic alternatives to Ellwood's magical uto-pian analysis. They chose not to listen.

During 1972 BCA, did various concrete things to mobilize the Plans. It held an HMO workshop at its national marketing meeting. It devel-oped more action-oriented policy guidelines to help encourage Plans to implement the HMO policy statement (BCA, 1972b). It published a very thorough manual on prepaid group practice development and operations (done with technical support from the Chicago Blue Cross Plan's HMO project staff) distributed copies nationwide, both inside and outside the Blue Cross system (BCA, 1972a). This was designed to make visible BCA's public interest leadership role.

The final 1972 development was a speech by Professor Robert Eilers, an internationally known authority on American health insurance, to Blue Cross Plan actuaries. He ended 1972 on the same HMO note that the Blue Cross system had heard at the beginning of 1970: HMO initiative was a survival issue. He closed by suggesting that Blue Cross would be pru-dent to heed the warning of J. Henry Smith, president of the Equitable Life Assurance Society, who said: "Our companies will significantly 'stay in business' only by developing effective participation in the organized delivery of services, especially HMOs" (p. 63). Eilers warned Blue Cross executives that if the Plans failed to meet the public's demand for HMO options, they would not have a role in the national health insurance pro-gram that was generally perceived to be emerging in Washington.

1973: Policy Swashbuckling

Nineteen hundred seventy-three was a year of Blue Cross HMO progress within a pressured and paranoid context. The Federal HMO Law (Public Law 93-222) was signed by President Nixon on December 10, 1973. Over the years its passage had been in doubt. Falkson gives an ex-cellent review of the 1970–73 period of HMO legislative action: "If the administration had lost its enthusiasm for HMOs, the [health] industry was certainly not going to stick its neck out. Thus hospitals, physicians, health insurers, and related businesses began to turn away from HMOs after what had been an all-too-brief flirtation" (1980, p. 165). The Blue Cross Association moved against this negative tide. BCA's ADS project was beefed up with an expansion of its field forces team. These were consultants that visited Blue Cross Plans to provide ADS technical assistance (TA), to act as catalysts for local Plan HMO initiatives and maintain liaison with the Plans.

BCA announced a major policy initiative at a February 27 press conference; its press release headline read: "New Symbol Heralds New Era for Nation's Blue Cross Plans: 10-point program calls for closer consumer ties, broader benefits, greater control of health costs, further expansion into group practice" (BCA, 1973b). This was a major move to further reposition Blue Cross closer to the public, away from its provider constituents, the hospitals. The change in the famous Blue Cross logo sent a clear message: the AHA symbol was removed from the Blue Cross logo, replaced by a human figure. McNerney explained: "The human figure in our new symbol, in replacing the American Hospital Association seal we have used up to now, shows that the primary concern of the Blue Cross system is to serve the public" (Blue Cross Association, 1973b). Group practice was highlighted in the press conference. McNerney was giving his prepaid group practice bandwagon visibility and symbolically locating it very centrally in the new image of Blue Cross that he was projecting: as an organization in the midst of changing with changing conditions and needs.

Other positive HMO steps taken by BCA included a conference at the just-opened Rochester Blue Cross Plan prepaid group practice. Also, BCA completed (and paid for) an HMO marketing film, *A Healthy Choice*, that was jointly sponsored by GHAA. Finally, a week-long executive seminar on HMO development was conducted for Plan executives by the Wharton School of Business in Philadelphia.

Despite these accomplishments, 1973 had more than an undercurrent of anxiety and paranoia. McNerney's annual report (BCA, 1973a) captured the anxious Watergate mood and a public demand for institutional renewal. He noted that "NHI will key off an economic model.... The country will buy neither egalitarianism nor elitism." He cited Philadelphia to illustrate the local politics of HMO development. There community groups were trying to put Blue Cross Plans in a subordinate role, while seeking key resources such as capital, risk management, marketing, and management from the Blues. His point about the touchy Blue Cross Plan—community advocacy group dynamics points at an irony. McNerney's many self-fulfilling prophecy tactics to create a Blue Cross

HMO bandwagon worked better with Blue Cross critics than with Blue Cross Plans. Critics believed McNerney's HMO bandwagon and saw the unruly, slow to innovate Blue Cross confederacy as a monolithic giant poised to take over the fledgling HMO field. Sylvia Law (1974) for example, wrote: "Blue Cross and other insurers have in fact moved to control and profit from HMO development.... On the national level, the BCA has encouraged the promotion of HMOs and made efforts to dispel criticism of Blue Cross dominance of HMOs" (p. 110). Still, she had a valid point. Many Blue Cross plans would launch HMO efforts within the stifling context of a traditional organizational culture. As Selznick suggests (1983): "The fear is that the character of the old organization will create resistance to the full development of the new program" (p. 41).

As dramatic as the press release's content was, the staging of the New York City press conference where it was delivered by McNerney was even more dramatic. For McNerney had kept most of his staff and his board in the dark about his HMO comments at the upcoming press conference. He used the press conference as a prod to stimulate Blue Cross action on HMOs. Without Board approval he predicted Blue Cross' HMO future: "By 1980 a total of 280 to 300 programs, are projected, covering an estimated seven million Blue Cross subscribers and their dependents." One vice president at BCA at the time recalls the press conference: "I'll never forget it because [McNerney] didn't tell anybody that he was going to say that [about 280 HMOs]. He didn't tell his board. He just said it to the press. It's a beautiful strategy when you think about it. What he was trying to do was *spark* the subject." The policy "goal" of 280 HMOs was used by McNerney as policy as prod. It was not as quantitative objective to be used seven years later for evaluation. Rather, it was used to "spark" action in the present.

This brings us back to the politics of institution building. As Selznick wrote, the opportunity to be a *creative* leader "depends on a considerable sensitivity to the politics of internal change. This is more than a struggle for power among contending groups and leaders. It is equally a matter of avoiding recalcitrance and releasing energies" (1983, p. 153). Leadership, for Selznick, *"is a kind of work done to meet the needs of a situation"* (p. 22). Moreover, situations are not given, but are continually interpreted and defined. They combine potentialities and limits. The leader has to be sensitive to the situation, able to grasp it. Interacting with his emerging definition of the situation is an emerging self-conception. As he comes to define a promising role for his institution to adopt, he is also adopting his role in and around the institution. This is so because role-taking "is in effect a decision by the individual...regarding how he ought to work. And this involves an estimate of his own place among others, including the demands placed upon him and his own capabilities" (p. 84). By *exploring possibilities* open to him, a leader begins to understand the constructive role he can play within the context of his social situation and own personality. Leadership, then is a dramatic exploration of the possible.

Moreover, the role-taking leader combines, according to Selznick, a will to act and a will to know. This recalls the formula "He who knows and communicates—controls." Communication—publicity or rhetoric— is a form of action. McNerney had interpreted the situation to which Blue Cross had to adapt. He decided that a prepaid group practice role was essential for a reinvented Blue Cross identity. He assessed his institutional context and decided that he could best release Blue Cross energy by *asserting* Blue Cross commitment—again, an anxious organization needs to declare itself The role he chose for himself to accomplish this was acting like a "swashbuckler." A BCA executive recalls:

> Walt has a couple of favorite phrases he uses. One is "swashbuckling." When I think of "swashbuckling" I think of Errol Flynn jumping off a pirate ship. I think Walt's approach in these [HMO] matters was to intellectually see the value of the thing. But he also knew he had a loose confederation of slow-moving people. How then, do you take what you're intellectually convinced in your own mind to be important to do, and get it done within that framework. His way of doing it was to be a swashbuckler. To call a press conference in New York, tell the world, and then suffer the consequences when he got back to his board.

McNerney periodically played the swashbuckling role to advance Blue Cross' development. (This was, of course, precisely John Mannix' style when he pushed for an American Blue Cross system. Correspondingly, it scared many local-based Blue Cross executives.) Whereas Benjamin Franklin, the ultimate role player, adopted his famous "strategic humility"— here we see McNerney adopting "tactical swashbuckling." McNerney played the swashbuckler at the New York press conference to goad his confederacy into action. When he got back to face his board "it was up in arms." An executive at the meeting recalls the flavor of the exchange:

> *McNerney:* "Yeah, I did that but you understand, I was just promoting the notion of Blue Cross..."
>
> *Board:* "Well yeah, but don't you think..."

McNerney: "Because...the market...you guys understand..."

Board: "Well, I don't know..."

Gradually he got them to go along with the idea.

He saw his statesmanship role occasionally needing some tactical swashbuckling in order to see that what the statesman designs "becomes a living reality" (Selznick, 1983 p. 37). Similarly, he tried to argue that BCA board members should serve the public and not organized medicine. He turned back his board's objections. Now the Blue Cross confederation had publicly tied itself to the goal of 280 HMOs by 1980. Still, he was leading a very reluctant constituency.

McNerney, then, shifted his limited ADS resources to a new division dedicated to containing health care costs. The new ADS Department was the bumptious crew that would, in swashbuckling style, swarm over ossified Blue Cross Plans and medical societies. It was of necessity a small department because the Board, still influenced by organized medicine, would not tolerate a full-fledged war on the status quo. The BCA HMO Strategy then was something more than the 1960s silent conspiracy to float the idea, but less than a full multiplier effect. It was an expedition into the possible today, to pave the way for full success in the 1980s.

1974–1977: A Pragmatic Approach to HMO Building

The period of 1973–1977 were years of HMO policy improvisation at the Blue Cross Association. I do not use "implementation" here because that word goes more with policy as plan. A master plan gets implemented, but policy as prod gets *improvised*. Schon (1971) calls this "a public learning system" (p. 116) which respects the potential of local regions to adapt general federal policy "themes" (p. 160)—and resources—to solve local problems. As a pragmatic approach, public learning systems assume that there is not one model that will fit all regions. Hence central policy is "*inductively* derived from the regions" (p. 160). So-called policy "implementation" is, then, actually local processes of social invention. Schon writes: "Central may provide first instances or policy themes which are take-off points for chains of transformation in localities. It may help local agencies to learn from one another's experience. It may even lend its weight to shifts in power structure which seem likely to lead to social discovery at the local level" (p. 161). This is a useful way to characterize the BCA approach to HMO action for this mid-1970s period: it was an improvising public learning system. McNerney's 1970 policy statement articulated a general theme. The subsequent Blue Cross national conferences gave Blue Cross executives some first instances or examples of this theme. Thus 1973 to 1978 were years of networking these executives to share lessons learned and to help facilitate local institution building. This facilitative role was built around a specific model of cooperative community HMO planning.

Before turning to the BCA facilitative phase of institution building it will be instructive to look at the parallel federal effort for these same years in terms of organization theory. Dr. Ellwood's HMO Strategy was based on Adam Smith's rational model of classical economics. Lyles and Thomas (1988) describe the characteristics of such rational models. The rational model stresses facts and optimal decision-making and excludes consideration of power, fear, and uncertainty. It does not regard problem formulation—defining the situation—as problematic. Ignoring problem formulation, however, can lead to "wishful thinking" (Lyles & Thomas, p. 135) i.e., utopian flights of fancy. Brown (1983) identifies precisely these shortcomings in his analysis of federal HMO strategy. The Ellwood policy analysis hid the complexities of the American health care system. As Brown observes: "Instead of pushing forward major operational issues for deliberation, it prevented them from being recognized as problematic" (p. 144).

Brown (1983) suggests that a proper model of HMO institution building should instead reveal "the opportunities and difficulties that attend the formation of HMOs" (p. 18). Brown offers a model of institution building based on the classical organization theory of Chester Barnard (1938) to describe an "HMO as a system of contributions" (Brown, 1983, p. 31). Brown argues that the federal HMO policy model hid the reality that HMOs are "complex" organizations (p. 31) that are hard to create. He uses Barnard's theory of the organization to show why it is hard to build an HMO. This is quite useful in explaining why many HMOs were *not* created.

Barnard's model is, however, less useful in helping us understand how many HMOs were built. This is so because Barnard's model is an "avoidance model" (Lyles & Thomas, p. 136) which is based on the conservative idea that organizations seek to avoid uncertainty and to preserve the status quo. Indeed, executives under this model will avoid perceiving a problem because the very existence of an emerging problem implies that leaders and followers alike are not doing their jobs properly. The hope is that if problems can be ignored long enough they will just go away. And indeed Brown characterizes the local HMO building process as an uncertain anxiety-provoking and professional reputation-threatening process. Hence, when, as is the case under Barnard's model, HMO developers do a "benefit-cost calculus," (Brown, 1983, p. 74) they often decide not to do anything.

Still, as Brown notes, hundreds of HMOs were started in the 1970s. This required people with "political skills," (1983, p. 88) "economic adeptness," "localistic insights," and "negotiating ability" (p. 89). These decisive people were not the risk adversive ones of Barnard's model, but rather action-oriented entrepreneurs. So we need a model of organization that is not built around a utilitarian accountancy of costs and benefits, but around a Deweyan drama, the exploration of the possible. In organization theory, the relevant model to describe successful HMO institution building is the "decisive organization" (Lyles & Thomas, p. 138). Here the actor thrives on uncertainty. The actor assumes that the situation is defined differently by people with competing attitudes. Given this uncertainty and competition to define the situation, the actor does not focus on making a rational optimal decision, nor does he or she hope that the situation will go away if avoided. Rather the actor—*acts*, that is, tries something. The outcome sought is not a perfect solution or a preserved status quo. Rather it is a "new situation" (Lyles & Thomas, p. 133)—a possibility explored.

Brown's assessment of the prospects for HMO institution building raises the Deweyan social learning possibility when he writes: "Health maintenance organizations are not machines to be assembled by master plan with interchangeable parts; rather they are artifacts in need of careful handcrafting" (Brown, 1983, p. 74). His study focuses on the federal HMO effort of the 1970s. He notes that Blue Cross plans and other insurers were the leading HMO sponsors in this period and that as the learning process "stumbled along," some insurance-sponsored plans surmounted their early difficulties and thrived (1983, p. 45). What I am suggesting here is that the Blue Cross confederation's HMO building learning process, for all its ups and downs, did not completely "stumble along," but was partially organized as a learning system, with the Association playing the facilitator role.

In 1974 the Blue Cross Association's HMO effort formalized its HMO policy follow-up by creating a new Alternative Delivery Systems Department, headed by Michael E. Henry. By this point thirty Plans were involved with over fifty ADS programs around the country. This new unit registered a shift in emphasis. Whereas earlier, the BCA emphasis had been educational with limited capacity to assist Plans in starting HMOs, that emphasis would now be revised. While continuing the educational function, now the emphasis was on facilitating Blue Cross Plans in specific HMO building activities.

The approach taken was a learning one, that is, to stress "lessons learned" by Blue Cross Plans already experienced in HMO ventures, to share this knowledge throughout the Blue Cross system, and to realistically identify common opportunities and "pitfalls" in most HMO planning situations (Henry, 1974). These are precisely the things found missing in the Federal strategy by Brown. Moreover, the approach stressed the role of local creativity in the process: "The ADS consulting approach is to put the HMO experience of the Blue Cross system into generalizable form. Still, each Blue Cross Plan is unique and is located in a unique environment. ADS will work with all interested Plans in adapting general principles to local circumstances" (Henry, 1974, p. 1). Henry, a natural pragmatist, improvised a social learning approach with a stress on building local institutions to fit the unique characteristics of particular locales. This is what Brown says was called for: handcrafted institution building. It also echoes the CCMC's pragmatic strand.

The ADS Department's action plan included several things to support its technical assistance role. First was its national HMO information service designed by staffer Johanna Sonnenfeld, which put out an ADS newsletter and HMO library. The information unit also held annual conferences that showcased exemplary instances of Blue Cross Plan HMO involvement. Second was project development that I headed that developed technical assistance and other relevant materials. Third were periodic workshops that acted as "a vehicle for sharing experience, communications, common problems/solutions and needs" (Henry, 1974, p. 8).

One tool helping to unite the various elements above was *A Guide to HMO Cooperative Planning* which I wrote (Miller, 1974). This Blue Cross approach to local HMO institution building rose out of "lessons learned" by the prepaid group practice movement (including that of Blue Cross Plans), was then put into published form for widespread distribution. It was the focus of a 1975 workshop. Also, it helped give coherence to ADS technical assistance efforts.

The Blue Cross Association's approach to HMO planning was premised on HMOs both having cost-containment potential and their being a "true *alternative* delivery system...competing with existing health care plans and providers, and maintaining an inherent competitive yardstick for the measurement of relative cost, quality and organizational effectiveness" (Miller, 1974, p. 1). Here were McNerney's two dimensions of ADS significance: as an option in the marketplace and also as an alternative format that would help discipline the dominant system. The mention of a "yardstick" was based on the example of the Tennessee Valley Authority (TVA). Picking up on both McNerney's and Henry's pragmatic stress of learning from experience, the cooperative approach to HMO planning was based on the forty-year experience of the prepaid group practice movement. Practical accounts of this experience (e.g., MacColl, 1966) warned readers of common problems in planning these alternatives. Similarly, Henry had stressed avoiding pitfalls in the planning process. Consequently, the cooperative approach "identified pitfalls...and promising approaches" (Miller, 1974, p. 3).

The cooperative approach emphasized that while there were exemplary HMO models and a common approach to the planning process, the key was in orchestrating the interaction of local "actors" in applying these historical models and general principles "to local circumstances" (Miller, 1974, p. 5). The HMO social learning process was driven by the "community situation" (p. 5). *The Guide* stressed that its approach "must be adjusted and particularized to fit needs and resources of each unique community" (p. 6). The approach set out within the *Guide* was not designed to represent a totally new way of thinking about what to do in planning HMOs, but rather, consolidated lessons already learned, and made explicit known pitfalls and effective principles, tools, and tactics—in an orderly and pragmatic way.

My own experience and readings shaped the *Guide*'s approach. My direct HMO planning experience had been an involvement in the late 1960s and early 1970s with one of the country's first HMO projects—that sponsored by a community organization in Chicago's Hyde Park-Kenwood neighborhood. First, as a neighborhood volunteer I worked on the Hyde Park-Kenwood Community Conference's healthcare task force. At the time I was a graduate student at the University of Chicago, studying political and social theory with Hannah Arendt. Then, after returning from Chapel Hill with an MPH in health policy and administration, I became the Task Force's HMO project director. After I joined BCA in late 1973, I continued my Hyde Park involvement serving as a board member of the developed operational community health center which was a contractual delivery point for citywide HMOs.

The BCA HMO approach also incorporated Dave Stewart's practical suggestion to "building on existing resources in the community while striving towards realizing the potential of fully integrated HMO systems" (Miller, 1974, p. 7). The *Guide* stressed Deweyan elements such as "actors," "action principles," and "interaction" (pp. 7-9). It tried to mediate between conservative incremental and radically totalistic planning approaches. It was a "strategic" approach in its stress on actors and interaction, on selectivity, and on avoiding "known pitfalls" (p. 9). The *Guide* stressed that HMOs are complex interorganizational coalitions: "An HMO...is an inter-organizational partnership among consumers, providers and managers, which focuses on the delivery of health care...HMOs [are] complex systems whose effective operation involves developing effective inter-organizational relationships" (Miller, 1974, pp. 10-11). Brown (1983) later made a similar observation. Crucial to the *Guide's* approach was its argument that HMO builders needed to be able to have a conceptual framework or attitude that let them see the problems and opportunities involved in the task. While seeing the potential of a managerial outlook it also, like Levine, warned about this outlook's shortcomings such as excessively impersonal patient care.

The cooperative approach meant "approach" not in the sense of a method of problem solving, but as a process of making *proposals*, of making *overtures* to begin relationships and move toward common courses of action. It was structured by Schein's (1969) concept of process consultation and its role in organization development. Schein's theory followed the social learning precepts of Lewin and Dewey. To this the *Guide* added power politics insights from international negotiations (Miller, 1974).

Schein (1969) stressed the importance of the definition of the situation and its relationship to role. He wrote: "The definition of the situation goes beyond specifying the goals or task to be achieved. It is the complete set of perceptions pertaining to one's own and others' roles in the situations, its duration, its boundaries and the norm that will govern it" (p. 27). His stress was on facilitating a process. He described some basic problems in group formation. They dealt with issues of identity, power, individual needs and group goals, and mutual acceptance. Understanding how group process unfolds, its problems, allows a facilitator to cope with the normal anxieties that arise in the group over these issues.

With respect to the kinds of problems Schein identified in group process, van Steenwyk described the following considerations in HMO inter-group planning (quoted in Miller, 1974, pp. 28–29). These are basic institution building points:

- The different HMO operating groups are likely to have different approaches, ideologies, operational methods, and clientele;
- each organization requires a degree of organizational autonomy (and that is valid);
- each can be effective (or at least is most likely to be) if the others give it an appropriate degree of support and recognition of its competence throughout the planning process—as this competence grows and is increasingly demonstrated;
- each partner will want to preserve in some fashion its identity (all deserve credit for their contributions to program viability);
- each will want a responsible and continuing role;
- the partners involved in such cooperative ventures each need to define its role and expectations in light of what it knows of the likely behavior and position of the others;
- there are real issues of power that at the appropriate time in the planning process need to be explicitly dealt with, and negotiated. In some cases the initial agreements may be less than perfect "partnerships," or may perhaps be reasonable accommodations; and
- facing the key issues of role negotiation can save much time and energy.

Such role development considerations are consistent with the assumption that community environments will often be active, characterized by many groups being concerned with HMO establishment and operation.

The cooperative approach matrixed these process considerations in which three categories of actors—manager, consumer and provider—interacted with the various technical dimensions of HMO planning such as finance, marketing, and so on. Its stress was on leaders from each group developing proposals and then working these through a process of negotiation. It explicitly built in the kinds of considerations that Brown (1983) later found lacking in the Federal strategy. Most of these were placed in a pre-feasibility phase called role *exploration* (Miller, p. 30). This is where, in our framework, possibilities were explored:

> The ADS coordinator must be familiar with the local environment, including both the medical and consumer communities. Crucial are group process skills.... The

ADS coordinator next explores for opportunities, support and barriers.... The ADS coordinator must strive to present and support the version of the concept which best fits his community's situation.... The ADS coordinator must seek a leader in each HMO interested actor or group with whom to coordinate inter-partner activity. Leadership is essential in HMO planning.... In determining provider and consumer implications, it is important to adequately identify consumer and provider allies and opponents.... Mutual education will need to take place. (Miller, 1974, pp. 30-35)

In his account of why the Federal HMO initiative led to the creation of relatively few HMOs in the 1970s, Brown quotes Rousseau approvingly: "The architect, before building a large edifice, studies and probes the ground it is to occupy, to find out whether it is capable of supporting so great a weight. The wise legislator, similarly, starts out not by drafting laws in and of themselves, but rather by finding out whether the people for whom he intends them is capable of bearing them" (Brown, 1983, p. 401). My point is that policy as prod includes preparing the ground, that is, a process of mutual education or social learning. This is Selznick's final point about creative leadership: to reconstruct the situation so that what is not possible today will be possible tomorrow. The Blue Cross HMO cooperative planning approach stressed precisely this pre-feasibility step. This is an essential step in social architecture properly understood. This "overture" step is analogous to Benveniste's "floating" of a utopian idea.

1975–1980

The 1975-80 period was characterized by a slow, steady widening of Blue Cross Plan HMO involvement, and it was also marked by doubts and hesitations. In 1975, twenty-eight Plans were involved with operational HMO programs (BCA, 1975a). By January of 1980 this had increased to forty-five Blue Cross Plans with HMO involvement. Although the Federal HMO Act had been passed in 1973, it was not until October of 1975 that the law's regulations concerning "dual choice" were finally issued (*ADS Coordinator*, November 4, 1975). These dual choice guidelines spelled out the conditions under which employers were mandated to offer federally approved HMOs to their employees. This was the belated "demand" side of the HMO Act. The lack of these regulations had stifled much potential demand for the new generation of 1970s HMOs. Also 1974-1975 featured an overall "stagflated," U.S. economy with both high inflation and unemployment rates—hardly the best of times to start small, innovative businesses such as HMOs. In a "blocked society" (Starr, 1982, p. 405), the Blue Cross Association's ADS Department nonetheless continued to stress community HMO leadership. It published HMO leadership guides for consumers, physicians, marketers, actuaries, and lawyers in 1975 and 1976.

McNerney in his 1975 Annual Report to his Blue Cross confederation, while keeping up his advocacy for Plan HMO involvement, added a new stress on the need for hooking up Blue Cross HMOs into a nationwide marketing network to efficiently meet the needs of national accounts. Big auto companies, for example, have employees in dozens of states which might involve scores of HMOs. A national network would hook these up so that a nationwide employer such as G.M. could deal with one Blue Cross Plan that would make a coordinated offer on behalf of the relevant HMOs.

In 1976 McNerney raised the additional issue of what he called "new directions." This was the newly emerging social criticism that challenged the assumptions that health services and health were identical, that the more services delivered, the healthier the population would get. Ivan Illich's *Medical Nemesis* (1976) was the lightning rod for much of the debate swirling over this issue (Star, 1982). The very phase "*heath maintenance organization*" raised this new doubt about the link between health status and health care services. *Could* an organization maintain people's health?

While more Blue Cross Plans tested the HMO waters, many did so out of defensive motives (Doherty, 1990). Still, a positive argument was formulated that saw Blue Cross HMO efforts as mediating change. John van Steenwyk, who consulted with a variety of clients including union pension and welfare funds, community sponsored HMOs, and the Blue Cross Association made the case that HMOs were not a federal spending fad but were an example of what the American health care system was evolving into (1975a). He argued to a Blue Cross audience: "As a nation, we need HMOs—not only for what they do, but also as examples and standard setters. While it is totally unrealistic to think of all health care as being delivered through HMOs, they are important beyond their numbers...as alternatives and examples" (1975b).

Van Steenwyk was pointing to the other aspects of policy besides "plan." HMOs were changing how people thought about health care ("perspective"), were examples of new ways of doing things ("prod"), and were alternatives that challenged the status quo ("position"). Eight years later

Brown (1983) made a similar case for HMOs. HMOs in the 1970s made, he suggests, a significant contribution beyond merely delivering some services and winning a bit of market share. They, as a form of institution building, "were catalytic or speculative in purpose, aiming to *trigger* 'system change'" (Brown, 1983 p. 433, italics added). As examples and alternatives 1970s HMOs "emboldened government, challenged the prevailing system and advanced a public philosophy of change" (Brown 1983, p. 493). Van Steenwyk and Brown were both making a "trigger phase" argument.

In 1976 BCA's Health Care Services got a new vice president, Neil Hollander. His job was to implement the cost containment policy formulated by Howard Berman, his predecessor. Hollander's implementation strategy was to institutionalize the various cost containment tactics or tools such as utilization review, area-wide health planning and ADS/HMO development by translating these recommended activities into BCA Board-approved mandatory Plan performance standards (Hollander, 1990). With respect to ADS policy, he crafted a standard that member Blue Cross Plans had to have an operational HMO in place or explain why not in writing both to their own boards and to BCA. The Blue Cross Association had traditionally used performance standards as a principal means of self-regulation. Plans had to subject themselves to self-study and external review by BCA staff, plus live with fishbowl peer pressure when their performance would be compared to national standards and averages. For cost containment, Hollander added the positive pressure of annual awards by the BCA Board to Plans for excellent cost containment performance, plus activity was guided by a special and prestigious blue ribbon subcommittee of the board.

Hollander makes a social learning case for the effectiveness of these tactics—they *prodded* plans into, for example, HMO action: "It helped in stimulating knowledge and response and gave leverage to those people in Plans who wanted to get something done. I don't know that BCA caused HMOs to be created, but we legitimized and *prodded* HMO development in some of the [Blue Cross] Plans. It may have been like pouring yeast into water and flour—a catalytic agent" (1990, italics added). This is pretty much the same argument that van Steenwyk and Brown used above to explain the significance of HMOs on the whole health care system. So the argument has two levels. The health care system, including Blue Cross Plans, had to be prodded into incremental HMO building—then HMOs would prod the system to evolve as a whole.

In 1977 the Carter administration rediscovered HMOs and began to promote them as standard-setters, as performance yardsticks (*ADS Coordinator*, July 1977). If, as Starr (1982) argues, the 1970s started by discovering the health care "crisis" and then in its middle years crisis became muddled into confusion, the end of the 1970s featured a major stress on competition in liberal and conservative thought and also on cooperation by the health care field. Carter's chief economic advisor, Charles Schultz (1977), suggested that marketplace competition be used to forward the public interest. Stanford economist Alain Enthoven developed a procompetition national health insurance model for Carter's HEW Secretary Joseph Califano (Starr, 1982). Meanwhile McNerney was reconstructing the old idea of "health care voluntarism." Voluntarism carried for him a sense of community-oriented action. In a major speech to a national convention of the hospital field, he said:

The word "voluntary" is...used to imply a level of pluralism, flexibility, and enterprise characteristic of local community effort.... Voluntary effort depends essentially on initiative that can be justified and given legitimacy only in terms of simple and direct dedication to public service, rather than formal legislative mandates or in response to the ingenious rules of the free marketplace. (McNerney, 1977, p. 58)

Here McNerney was reinventing the pragmatic social control idea, that is, that society, or part of it, could guide itself by balancing social forces—here government regulation, marketplace competition and community initiative (cooperation)—towards some public interest ideal (Janowitz, 1978). Like Janowitz (1978), McNerney's control force was social, not economic-based. And like Janowitz, McNerney put a pragmatic stress on local institution building. This local initiative had, however, to be coordinated with federal policy themes. McNerney cautioned that: "It requires a high degree of wisdom and sophistication to see the solution of national problems in the form of separate but interrelated local initiatives; national initiatives on the surface seem neater and more appealing" (McNerney, 1977, p. 62). He also issued a call for increased local health care action and innovation to build "viable community-based alternatives" (p. 74). This hinged on there being enough true Blue Cross and hospital leaders at the local level to inspire a social movement. Leadership in turn required people having a sense of mission. He flatly stated that without a sense of mission "voluntarism as we know it will be lost" (p. 73). He cited the words from a *South Pacific* song: "You gotta have a dream, if you don't have a dream, how you gonna have a dream come true?" Institution building requires spirit, that is, passion; therefore leaders must spell out utopian dreams.

Many in the audience did not know what to make of this call for a renewal of voluntary spirit; they had trouble grasping what he had in mind. He was challenging them to explore the possible with imagination and they were looking for a clear road map. One sophisticated health care consultant's response is illustrative: "I don't think Walt has been specific yet. What are the different financing mechanisms?" (Meyer, 1977, p. 56). This consultant did, however, astutely see the political complexity of community action, perhaps more fully than McNerney did at the time: "The notion of talking about how the providers get together to finance hospitalization is important, but we must also get together representatives from labor, business, management and government.... Unless we get all these people together I don't know" (Meyer, 1977, pp. 56–57).

Interestingly, the prime examples offered by people in the audience of McNerney's idea were HMOs. Finally, some in the audience asked if this call for "voluntarism" was just posturing for coming national health insurance (NHI). In the late 1970s, as the hospital industry faced the threat of the Federal government passing NHI legislation, it joined with Blue Cross and Shield in the "Voluntary Effort" (VE) to control health care costs. Although meant as a prod by McNerney to stir up community innovation and reform, VE quickly became simply a ploy to stall legislation. Once the prospects for the legislation dimmed, the VE initiative lost its momentum (Stevens, 1989). Moreover, Americans concerned about their health and mortality were not interested in restricting the growth of hospital services (Anderson, 1985).

The mix for much 1980s health care activity was foreshadowed in the late 1970s with its emerging cooperation and competition themes. One key mixture in the 1980s of these ingredients would be local groups cooperating to build competitive HMOs in hope of controlling health care costs. Overall, however, health care in America in the 1970s became increasingly commercialized (Stevens, 1989). "Voluntarism" had all but disappeared as a credible posture by the not-for-profit segment of American health care (Starr, 1982; Stevens, 1989) which turned more and more to the, to borrow Stuart's words, "moving lights from the near-by shore of expediency."

In 1978 the Blue Cross Association and Blue Shield Association merged their staffs in preparation for a merger of boards in 1982. The associations' two ADS departments were correspondingly merged under executives from the Blue Shield organization. The department's combined staff was subsequently cut in half. One strength of the new, low-key unit was that the old group practice vs. individual practice HMO debate between Blue Cross and Blue Shield staffs was now put aside. The new unit saw the two formats as more or less useful depending on local conditions.

The Blue Cross HMO movement had not yet passed what one former Blue Cross executive calls "the third threshold: where the majority of Blue Cross Plans crossed over the bridge from where HMOs were a defensive thing or something only to be meddled with, to the other side of the bridge where HMOs became a product line critical to the long term success of the Blue Cross movement." For this, he suggests, the movement had to wait for employers to truly demand HMOs. This "multiplier" came in the 1980s; so did the "contrary currents of commercial competition."

4

Consequences: Establishment and Organizational Character (1980s–1995)

The Heyday 1980s

George Will, the conservative columnist, summed up the 1980s this way: "The cheerfulness that has defined Reagan's era of good feelings has been on balance, salutary. But it also has been a narcotic, numbing the nation's senses about hazards just over the horizon" (1990, p. 141). He noted one hazard that has arrived: the tens of millions of Americans without health insurance. Another hazard was about to arrive: a Blue Cross Plan was soon to go bankrupt. Kevin Phillips (1990) another Republican pundit, pointed out that in Republican heyday periods, such as the Roaring Twenties and the Reagan 1980s, the growth in wealth is unevenly shared. Most goes to the economic elite. Ross Perot, who made his billion the old fashion way by developing a new service and a new company, criticized the gunslinger entrepreneur of the 1980s who made fortunes via junk bonds and S & L swindles. He noted that "now it's the taxpayer, the average citizen who's become the entrepreneur in fact, with all the risk and very little of the reward" (quoted in Phillips, p. 72). Soon, some Blue Cross Plans would sink into scandal.

Eli Ginsberg (1990) has argued that the Reagan administration had monetarized and destabilized American health care. In effect it did so by endorsing the medical industrial complex. In 1981 the administration announced that it would rely on competition, not regulation, to reform American health care. This procompetition vocabulary cloaked an "underdevelopment" (Whiteis & Salmon, 1987, p. 19) of public and voluntary sector health care. Reagan carried forward two ideas incubated in the Carter administration: Enthoven's idea of releasing competitive forces in health care and the federally financed DRG experiment in New Jersey.

Over the past fifteen years the legitimacy of the nonprofit ideology was severely eroded. This was prepared for in the 1960s and the 1970s. In the 1960s Medicare ironically encouraged nonprofit hospitals and Blue Cross Plans to behave in more commercial fashion (Stevens, 1989). In the 1970s the Nixon administration's HMO strategy opened the door for for-profit firms to establish alternative delivery systems. Also, its premises included doubt about the utility of government's role in health care and a utopian faith in both the marketplace and in economic incentives to shape individual and institutional behaviors. Voluntary and governmental faiths began to decline. The marketplace faith began to gain followers (Marmor, Schlesinger & Smithey, 1994). The voluntary ethic was being challenged by the spirit of capitalism.

Overall, the 1980s were shaped by the Reagan revolution which ideologically generalized on the 1970s premises that underlay the HMO strategy: social problems were best addressed by marketplace competition. Profits would fuel progress. This drained the voluntary nonprofit ideology of much of its legitimacy (Estes, 1994). Estes observes: "The attack on the nonprofit sector in health care is part of the...phenomena: new opportunities for corporate investment capital in health are needed and the opportunities for proprietaries in the health care market are enhanced with the weakening of the nonprofit sector and the erosion of its legitimacy (p. 145)."

Four Revolutions: Restructuring

Around 1980, after the Blue Cross and Shield trade associations merged their management in preparation for a 1982 merger of boards, McNerney (for the AHA oral history collection), shared his private reflections on Blue Cross' identity. He talked about what he called "the community idea" and "central conscience" (McNerney, 1984, p. 98). The "community idea" was what he called over the years, Blue Cross' North Star: its philosophical community service origins and direction. (This was the tradition of the conciliatory Rorem.) The "central conscience" referred to the need for some power to move to the national association to do certain business things more efficiently (represented by the swashbuckling Mannix). The community idea was a radical impulse that had been precariously stamped into Blue Cross' character. Mannix' radical vision of the Blues operating effectively as a national network serving national accounts had been resisted strongly by Blue Cross CEOs over the years.

With respect to the "centralizing concept," he thought that the associations could help develop products and provide improved uniformity of service to national accounts. He noted that his leadership at the Blue Cross Association had always been based on a powerful cohesive minority—what Pettigrew (1987) calls a "change caucus"—of a half-dozen plan CEOs who shared the community idea and some degree of central conscience. He noted ominously: "Today [1980] interestingly enough, five or six plan presidents with that type of zeal and conviction are still of critical importance. Some days I think I'm down to three" (McNerney, 1984, p. 118). He had failed to replenish his change caucus as retirement removed his key supporters. Moreover, he decided not to attempt to include non-Blue Cross Plan CEOs on the merged Association's board. Despite some indications that an HMO enrollment effect might be taking off such as a *Business Week* ("A Bright Prognosis," 1980, October 27) HMO article, HMO enrollment had not yet soared. He remarked, "Personally after twenty years as CEO, I should seek another career and make room for new blood—for my sake and for the corporation's" (1984, p. 115). Like Rorem, he was growing tired of trying to get his membership to properly function.

In 1981 came a board revolution. The board rejected McNerney's leadership themes of community and centralization. He clashed with his board and resigned. *Business Week* reported that he reigned because he could not prod his Plans "to modernize their operations or offerings" ("A Health Insurer That Needed a Cure," 1982, May 10). And there was still some deep resentment of McNerney's swashbuckling support of prepaid group practice and HMOs over the years. Finally, there was the irony that McNerney had been hired as a public spokesman/lobbyist to the federal government, but the 1980s were for the Blues going to be a local market-driven decade. He had lost federal pressure as a key lever in influencing his board. He had become dispensable.

McNerney suffered a fate not uncommon in America to leaders with community as their guiding consideration. As historian Robert Wiebe observes, "In the twentieth century, those few people who wanted their new occupational segments to influence a wide range of social issues declared themselves generals without an army. From Samuel Gompers to John L. Lewis to Walter Reuther, officials who tried to translate [narrow] loyalty into broad social objectives either failed and retreated or failed and retired" (Wiebe, 1975, p. 91). In a decade of greed, health care executives did not want to hear about a community service mission. This disregard for mission, however, carried with it a danger: loss of identity and integrity. Now many Plans turned towards profitmaking and perks, many interested in entrepreneurial means and too often ignoring community ends.

Still, as Sibery recalls, it was McNerney who argued in the 1970s that Blue Cross plans could only stem the loss of members and money by diversifying. He evaluates McNerney's leadership: "Had the Walt McNerney's of the world felt that the Blues could go on as they were with no change, I think it is questionable whether we would have meaningful impact in 1987 or not" (1987, pp. 33–34). McNerney had in the 1970s positioned the Blues so that they could be a factor in the 1980s health care market place.

In 1982 American health care purchaser attitudes changed and the HMO multiplier effect kicked in. This was a purchaser revolution. Ginsberg (1990) notes that the severe 1981–82 recession had tremendous impact on health care. This economic shock delivered what McNerney had wanted from government back in 1972: a big crunch to spur change. Eugene Sibery (1990) recalls that when he took over as Iowa Blue Cross' new CEO, he was on the job only two weeks when the heads of his plan's major accounts came into his office and announced that they wanted to see demonstrable change from the plan within three months or they would take their business—27 percent of the plan's enrollees—elsewhere. He observes that the early 1980s environment was totally different than in the previous decade—although few around the country realized it then. As *Business Week* ("The Spiraling Costs of Health Care," 1982, February 8) reported, employers were jumping onto the bandwagon to get some relief from skyrocketing health care costs. As Blue Cross and Blue Shield's traditional product lines were taking a battering, their HMOs offered them their only rays of hope. As Neil Hollander said, the Blues "no longer consider HMOs an experimental line of business. It's our bread and butter. It's our major growth in many parts of the country" (Iglehart, 1982, p. 453).

In 1980 and 1981 the Blue Cross and Blue Shield plans lost in the aggregate $889 million. *Business Week* ("A Health Insurer," 1982, May 10) suggested that the Blues "needed a cure." In 1982, Bernard Tresnowski succeeded McNerney as president of the now merged Blue Cross and Blue Shield Association. He admitted that the Blues were "humbled" ("A Health Insurer," 1982 May 10, p. 163) and argued that the experience readied his member plans for changes (Friedman, 1982). *Fortune* described 1982 this way:

> If there was ever a year for American industry to get serious about curbing the runaway cost of employer medical benefits, 1982 was it. While profits of the *Fortune* 500 were tumbling…the price index of health care surged another 11.6 percent. Many companies' medical insurance premiums jumped 20 percent…. Some top managements are at last looking for cures and finding at least partial relief. (Richman, 1983, p. 95)

Most big companies, Ginsberg (1990) observed, which had ignored the 1970s health care cost explosion were shocked in the early 1980s into action. They moved in several directions. Many left their health insurer and self-insured. This, Ginsberg notes, fractured the "risk pool" (p. 280), leaving the insurers with fewer and relatively sicker subscribers. Employers also began on a widespread basis to enthusiastically offer and advocate HMO options to their employees. The HMO mobilizer had come. Soon private insurers and for-profit hospitals were rushing to join with Blue Cross in the HMO market. Within the Blue Cross system HMOs were largely, but not universally accepted as crucial to Blue Cross survival.

Also in 1982, the *New York Times* conducted a national opinion poll asking Americans what they would give up if it would help contain health care costs. Strikingly, 50 percent of the people polled indicated that they would enroll in a prepaid group practices clinic ("Majority Would Change Health Coverage," 1982, May). Employees, then, were as ready as employers for alternative health care arrangements. By 1982 there were some seventy community health care coalitions around the nation, about 70 percent of which were involved with HMO development ("Majority of Business Coalitions," 1982, October). Also that year Virgil Marsh of BCBSA worked with the Chicago Blue Cross and Shield Plan to develop the first nationwide HMO network for a private account: United Airlines ("HCSC Introduced HMO Network," p. 1). In 1982 the Reagan administration published *The Investor's Guide To HMOs*. Its message: there was money to be made in HMOs. HMOs were now at the heart of the medical-industrial empire. Finally, in 1982 "the total number of people covered for hospital care through non-governmental sources peaked at 188 million" (AHA, 1990, p. 23). Along the way, Blue Cross' identity as a community-based social institution had become seriously eroded. In 1986 Blue Cross plans, for example, lost their federal not-for-profit tax exemption (Stevens, 1989). Interestingly, not-for-profit HMOs kept their tax-exempt status ("Non profit HMOs," 1986, April/May).

With Tresnowski came a product revolution. When in 1982 Bernard Tresnowski became the president of the Blue Cross and Blue Shield Association it was clear that his board wanted not a public-oriented health care statesman, but rather a market-oriented corporate executive who would mind the store and help save its bacon in the marketplace. As Selznick (1983) observed, a leader cannot simply shape the organization to fit his own personal values: "A wise leader faces up to the character of his organization, although he may do so only as a prelude to designing a strategy that will alter it" (p.70). Tresnowski found himself leading a confederation of Blue Cross and Shield Plans under attack in the market place. He felt that speeches about the public good would in this context be "utopian wishful thinking" to use Selznick's phrase (1983, p. 148), and he retreated from Blue Cross' community mission. Tresnowski's challenge was to consolidate the gains of McNerney's creative leadership in exerting a, again to use Selznick's language, "cohesive force in the direction of institutional security." Ironically, this involved three more Blue revolutions: product, governance, and policy. In the period of 1982–1987 the Association developed new HMO, PPO, and Managed Care alternatives to the traditional fee-for-service products.

In terms of the shifting rhetorical styles in a social movement—and some Blue Cross and Shield people once saw their enterprise this way (Anderson, 1975)—the McNerney-Tresnowski transition was from the reform rhetoric of a gadfly that marks the movement's "mobilization" stage (1984, Stewart, Smith & Denton, p. 43) to the managerial rhetoric of a leader in the "maintenance" (p. 44) stage. In a social movement's maintenance stage, membership and commitment declines. Money becomes the movement's driver "and the leader becomes an entrepreneur rather than a reformer. Routinization of dues, meetings, leadership, decision-making, and rituals seem essentials for a highly structured and disciplined movement [to] survive and carry the cause forward. These bureaucratic necessities, however, siphon off much of the old… *esprit de corps* that made the movement vibrant and attractive" (Stewart, Smith & Denton, p. 45). Eventually the maintenance phase either finds a way to "make the cause fun again" (Stewart, Smith & Denton, p. 45) or the movement dies.

While sharing McNerney's community service values, Tresnowski faced a different situation and had a different leadership style. Unlike McNerney who periodically would jump-start Blue Cross evolution with one swashbuckling challenge or another, Tresnowski was more of a slow consensus-builder. He was, like Rorem, more conciliatory. When McNerney's pedagogical mode was the "lecture," Tresnowski favored "group projects." Tresnowski organized his Blue Cross and Blue Shield Board so that they discovered things for themselves. In 1982 he quickly established a Board strategic planning task force to create a "Five Year Business and Diversification Strategy" (Blue Cross and Blue Shield Association, 1990). In doing so, he moved his rambunctious confederation down the high speed toll road of entrepreneurship that McNerney had opened. Under Tresnowski, the Blue Cross movement became commercialized.

The task force decided to diversify into things that would strengthen the core Blue Cross and Shield business. This led it to HMOs, PPOS, and so on. There were two problems. First was that diversification requires capital. So the task force recommended establishing Capital Service Corporation (CSC) which could attract capital and in turn invest it into new product development. The second problem was that national accounts did not want to deal separately with many Blue Cross/Shield HMOs around the nation. So the Task Force took BCA's 1970s national HMO network policy work and the 1982 ad hoc national HMO network for United Airlines and proposed a new product: HMO-USA (a national HMO network). Both CSC and HMO-USA have been successes. Tresnowski took what McNerney had done in terms of creating HMOs, found a capital source and found a vehicle to network the thing. BCA had such success with HMO-USA that it created Preferred Care-USA (a network of PPOS) and then Custom Care USA (a network of the various managed care tools that are applied to HMOs, PPOs, or fee-for-service policies).

Note that while the Plans had rejected McNerney's institution building themes of community and centralization, some were receptive to new produce lines. This repeats their deletion of the word "worthy" in the original HMO policy statement ten years earlier. The Plans always resisted institution building, but accepted new product lines when commercially necessary. So, what were radical reforms in the McNerney years, became (practically overnight) in 1982, expedient entrepreneurial moves at the start of the Tresnowski era. Where McNerney traumatized his board in 1973 by moving HMOs symbolically closer to the core of Blue Cross identity, Tresnowski about ten years later let his board move HMO diversification to the center of its survival strategy. Structure had followed symbol. Nationwide HMO enrollment began to rocket upwards in 1983 (Hale

& Hunter, 1988). From 1977 to 1982 HMO enrollment increased each year by about .7 million people. Then, in 1983 it jumped 1.7 million, in 1984 by 2.6 million, and so on. McNerney was proven correct as purchasers of health insurance defected from traditional products to HMO alternatives. But in the struggle for Blue Cross' soul, McNerney lost. He had looked to marketplace competition as a countervailing force to discipline voluntary and governmental excesses—but once unleashed, capitalism moved to become the prevailing force in health care.

By 1984 Tresnowski was speaking about Blue Cross' organizational mission in commercial terms of a "product portfolio"—community and centralization had receded (Tresnowski, 1985, p. 3). He highlighted the key role played by HMOs in this portfolio:

> Today, more than fifty thousand employers offer an HMO to their employees. The Blue Cross and Blue Shield Organization saw HMOs as a market opportunity, and we also saw HMOs as an important ingredient in putting the delivery system in order and in offering choices and options. Consequently, Blue Cross and Blue Shield have invested $100 million dollars in HMO development over the past 10 years. At the end of 1983, forty Blue Cross and Blue Shield plans were operating forty-seven HMOs in twenty-seven states.

> In 1983 alone we added seven new HMOs. Enrollment in Blue Cross and Blue Shield HMOs now exceeds 1.5 million members. In 1983, our growth in the HMO line of business was twenty-six percent, compared to a sixteen percent growth for HMOs generally. It is our fastest-growing line of business. In fact, it is our only growing line of business. (1985, p. 4)

In the 1980s some of the Blues were, then, reinventing themselves into HMO-like organizations—while still seeing themselves as financiers of health care. The Blues were, under Tresnowski's leadership moving backwards from McNerney's organizations—to institution direction. Now the Blues were beginning to shift back to becoming organizations without social values.

In the 1980s the health insurance market was reformulated. Coverage in managed care plans went from 1.5 percent of all group health coverage in 1982 to 72 percent in 1988 (AHA, 1990). Where approximately 26 million people lacked health insurance in 1978, by 1987 this had risen to approximately 37 million (AHA, 1990). Interestingly, the medical-industrial complex moved decisively into the HMO field, converting it into a profitable industry in the post-1982 years. In the 1985–1989 period, approximately 300 new for-profit HMOs entered the market, compared with approximately 90 new not-for-profit HMOs (AHA, 1990).

By 1985, the darker consequences of the medical-industrial complex— predicted by Health PAC, Robert Levine, Salmon and others—was surfacing. Robert Wiebe (1975) has observed that America rediscovers poverty about every thirty years. Suddenly our indifference is pierced and we rediscover the poor. In the self-centered 1980s many people with access to health care had an attitude not dissimilar to that expressed by Morris Fishbein years before: "A little sickness [in others] is not too great a price to pay for maintaining democracy" (quoted in Wiebe, 1975, p. 179). Then in the mid-1980s America discovered tens of millions of people without health insurance. One leader of the not-for-profit hospital field, Bruce Vladeck (1985), called for "a rededication to community service" (p. 115). He warned that hospitals would lose their legitimacy if they failed to serve their communities. As the loose Blue Cross and Shield confederation became entrepreneurial, plan adventurism eroded "central consciousness" as some Blue Cross and Shield Plans clearly challenged the Association's authority to license the names "Blue Cross" and "Blue Shield" to member Plans (Blue Cross and Blue Shield Association, 1987). Beneath the cover of the national Blue Cross image some plans were retreating into outdated understandings of their mission, while others were leaping to seize illusory future opportunities.

Although, Blue Cross and Blue Shield HMO enrollment from 1985 to 1989 rocketed from 2 million to 5 million, the confederation was in deep trouble. A *Business Week* (Deveny, 1988, Feb. 15, pp. 33–34) article headline summarized the situation: "What's Ailing Blue Cross...Competition, rising costs and poor management dog the insurer." In 1987 the confederation lost $800 million. Lack of nationwide product and service uniformity continued to aggravate Blue Cross and Shield customers. *Business Week* concluded by suggesting that HMO's were the cure for the confederation's problems, (1989, December 4).

From 1984 to 1988 Blue Cross and Shield plan enrollment in traditional fee-for-service health care policies declined from 76 million people to 38 million. Because of its alternative products such as HMOs, PPOs, and Managed Care, it was able to suffer a net loss of "just" 8 million people in this five-year period (Kirschner, 1989). Richard Maturi, BCBSA's executive director of managed care programs called the growth of Blue Cross and Shield alternatives "the product revolution" and noted that "the management revolution (at BCBSA) is going on right now" (Kirschner, 1989, p. 9).

Tresnowski believed that the health care cost, quality, and access problems would not be solved by ideological rhetoric, but by recognizing that we need to find ways to combine economic and clinical decision-making. He suggested that "the model for those decisions is the staff-model health maintenance organization. It combines delivery and finance into a single system. But you are never going to get widespread application of that. So instead we substitute selective interventions called managed care" (insider interview, 1989, December 4, p. 12).

The 1987–90 period constituted a management revolution characterized by "concern, debate, stress, and tension" (Blue Cross & Blue Shield Association, 1988, p. 20) for the BCBSA confederation as it struggled to find rules to govern itself cohesively in a turbulent market place. In 1987 the confederation began to debate the size, structure, and accountability of the Association's board. Using a format called the "Assembly of Plans"—a committee of the whole (of all Plans), Plan CEO's went through what Tresnowski called a "learning" (BCBSA, 1988, p. 18) process that was structured to lessen large Plan versus small Plan divisiveness. The hope, unforfilled, was that this process would be the confederation's constitutional convention—but it did not produce a more federal, that is, unified, system. In 1988 this Assembly of Plans process produced a new National Account Business Policy that for the first time in the confederation's history offered, they hoped, the prospect of a truly coordinated, collective approach to acquiring, service and retaining national accounts (BCBSA, 1989). Servicing national accounts, however, remained a major problem.

Tresnowski closed the 1980s by sharing his vision for the future with his colleagues: "The foundation of our vision should be the willingness and ability to do three basic things: to learn, to grow, and to change" (BCBSA, 1989, p. 27). These are social learning tradition core ideas. Interestingly, he, as befitting a leader of a movement deep in a money-driven maintenance phase, raised the issue of "fun": "Some have declared that our business has become so demanding that the "fun" has gone out of their jobs. I would assert that taking the opportunity to learn and grow and change will not only bring something new and positive to our work, it will add the enjoyment we all want to experience" (BCBSA, 1989, p. 27).

Haltingly, many Plans in the 1980s followed Tresnowski's vision of managed care. In this entrepreneurial push, some drifted away from "the community idea" and most continued to resist "a centralized conscience." Strikingly, the Assembly of Plans chose not to deal with reconstructing a common Blue Cross mission. Blue Cross had positioned itself for the 1990s managed care market, but its unique identity had become precarious.

1990: A Policy Revolution

America's health care situation in the 1990s is one of expensive desperation. Things looked bleak, for example, in the house of medicine. Dr. Richard Reece reported on his talks with a cross section of his colleagues: "Everywhere I hear uneasiness about the directions medicine is headed—the discounting of fees, demands for accountability, the disappearance of practitioners into organizations, the intrusion of managed care, the explosion of utilization review, the erosion of traditional values, physician-bashing by politicians and a decline of patient loyalty" (quoted in Anderson, O.W., 1990, p. 336). Sometimes patients blame physicians, pointing out that physician income rose from $90,000 in 1982 to $156,000 in 1989 (Jacobson, 1991, May 6, p. 1). Lost in this blame game was the fact that over 10 percent of health care costs were attributable to fraud ("Report: Health Fraud," *Chicago Tribune*, July 8, 1994, p. 11).

Meanwhile, Robert Laszewski, while Liberty Mutual Insurance Group's executive vice president, suffered an ever-increasing health consumer nightmare: having a seriously ill family member, needing extensive rehabilitative services, whose health plan stopped paying claims long before that relative had regained her health (Millenson, 1991, July 10). Indeed a new specter haunts middle-class America: becoming one of the health care uninsured. As the *New York Times*' Tamar Lewin put it:

> Long a gnawing worry of the poor, medical expenses and health insurance are now a source of mounting anxiety for millions of middle-class Americans—healthy or sick, insured or not. For a growing number of people, insurance status has become the pivotal factor in important personal decisions, trapping some people in jobs [to keep their insurance] and forcing others to forego needed medical treatment. (1991, April 4, p. 1)

By 1990 the health insurance marketplace was destroying itself with hyper-entrepreneurship. As Robert Laszewski noted, the increasing practice of insurers shedding rather than sharing risks—for example, dropping people who file large claims—is "a classic example of an industry courting suicide" (Wasik, 1991, p. 58). The 1980s played out like a tragic repeat and reversal of the 1950s when commercial insurers and their indemnity practices entered the health insurance market dominated then by Blue Cross and Blue Shield. But while in the 1950s the number of people covered by health insurance greatly increased, in the 1980s it was the number of uninsured that skyrocketed. HMOs in their competitive and venture capitalism garb provided by the Nixon and Reagan administrations contributed to this commercial trend.

Just as Blue Cross and Shield Plans in the 1960s had to partially convert from their traditional community rating method to the commercials' experience rating approach, in the 1980s HMOs were forced to do the same thing (Hale & Hunter, 1988). As Hale and Hunter observe, HMOs originally had a consumer-oriented organizational character but this was eroded as "HMOs compete with and adopt characteristics of their insurance-like competitors.... Community rating, designed to offer the most affordable coverage to the broad population, has largely been supplanted by experience rating and competition for the best risks" (p. 48).

Consumer Reports concluded, for example, that the Blue Cross and Blue Shield confederation had abandoned its community service mission, becoming more and more like commercial insurers ("The Crisis," August, 1990). As other insurers cease to be risk sharers and become risk shedders (Wasik, July, 1991), Blue Cross is forced to abandon its mission or go out of business. Indeed, *Consumer Reports* observes that often it is state regulators that encourage Blue Cross and Blue Shield Plans to drop community rating and re-incorporate as mutual insurance companies.

In this destructive vortex of a health insurance market place, Tresnowski tried to convince his member Plans not to overly imitate their commercial competitors. Consequently, having successful product and governance revolutions, he shifted to a policy statesperson role. Where McNerney had allied the Blues with the federal government, Tresnowski allied them with the largest for-profit health insurance companies—he joined the Jackson Hole health reform group. He worked with Congressional leaders to have Congress consider proposals to reform the health insurance industry in a managed care and managed competition format. Similarly, the *New York Times* editors also pushed for reforms that would prohibit insurer risk shedding:

> The best answer is a system known as managed competition under which every individual would be part of a large group. A sponsor, probably a large employer or government agency, would solicit bids from private insurers, which would be required to offer coverage to everyone at uniform rates. Nor would insurers be allowed to cancel policies of people who became chronically ill. ("Don't Blame Blue Cross," Aug. 12, 1991, p. A14)

Ironically, as Tresnowski tried to get the confederation to become less defensive inside, it became more defensive externally. As the Plans united further together in turning out new products to sell, they separated more and more from each other and their traditional common community mission. They denied the public information. Blue Cross and Blue Shield Plans were, as in the 1970s, becoming contumacious, that is, resistant to accountability and regulation. As one state insurance regulator put it: "We think the Blues in our state do a pretty good job. But everyone here dislikes them.... They are some of the most defensive people you can imagine. Everything we ask for is a fight" ("The Crisis in Health Insurance," 1990, August, p. 553). Strikingly, of twenty-nine Blue Cross and Shield Plans that *Consumer Reports* asked to cooperate in a comparative analysis of various health insurance companies, only nine agreed to provide copies of their benefit policies ("The Crisis in Health Insurance"). For all the *perestroika* (restructuring) that the confederation had done in the 1980s, it had rejected *glasnost* (publicity) when it came to providing agents of the public with information about its products. The Blues had begun to act as if they had something to hide. How can the consumer and the public learn, grow, and be open to change if Blue Cross and Blue Shield do not share facts with them? How can managed competition work if the Blues won't share basic product information with consumer organizations such as *Consumer Reports*? In the 1980s and early 1990s, many Blue Cross Plans made critical decisions that had basic consequences for their organization's character.

Irresponsible Leadership

In 1990 a Blue Cross and Blue Shield plan—one in West Virginia—failed. This was the first time a Blue Plan had ever become bankrupt. The Association was fairly passive in holding the West Virginia Plan to its membership standards; nor did the Association have the financial means to protect the Plans subscribers. As the *Wall Street Journal* observed, the Association "is mainly a public-relations and lobbying body without financial resources of its own" (Pulliam, March 8, 1991, p. 17). In 1991 the U.S. Senate's Permanent Subcommittee on Investigations began a three-year inquiry into what went wrong there and the possibility of potential Blue Cross and Blue Shield failures elsewhere. These investigations raised the issue of a Blue Cross identity crisis. John Sopko, deputy chief counsel to the Subcommittee noted, at its July 2, 1992 hearing, a widely perceived shift in the organizational character of Blue Cross plans across the nation—many plans had become commercialized and contumacious, that is, had become profit-seeking in the market place and resistant to authority in the public realm. He noted that this character change had let the National Association of Insurance Commissioners to form a new committee to focus on fiscal and accountability problems with Blue Cross and Blue Shield plans. He cited John Danaho's (a member of the Association and recent insurance commissioner of Maryland until removed from his position for being too critical of the Blues) list of Blue Cross problems: "(1) generally poor and inexperienced management; (2) failure to accept regulation and a desire to subvert it; (3) involvement in subsidiary operations without prior notice, sometimes inconsistent with their primary mission and in violation of insurance regulation and orders; (4) insolvency; (5) failure to keep insurance commissioners informed of their problems; (6) strange attempts to influence administration and legislative policy making; (7) poor public relations, both to subscribers and providers; (8) incompetent claims management and late payments; and (9) no apparent attempt to cost control or operating efficiency" (U.S. Senate, July, pp. 6–7).

Sopko was quick to point out that while there were several Blue Cross and Blue Shield Plans that seemed to merit investigation on these counts, the investigation had *no* evidence that "the vast majority of the Blues are not being run in a proper and fiscally sound manner" (p. 7). Still, he noted that the staff did not have a paucity of Plans to investigate. He went on to list some of the apparent management abuses that were alleged. They included:

- a Blue Cross/Blue Shield Plan paying its CEO $350,000 a year plus country club memberships and a chauffeur-driven limousine plus a $1.2 million pension buyout arrangement while the Plan is nearly insolvent;
- a Blue Cross/Blue Shield Plan giving a construction contract to its chairman of the board of directors even though this construction contract was not the lowest bid;
- two Blue Cross/Blue Shield Plans purchasing sky boxes at local stadiums while at the same time requesting extensive rate increases due to problems with costs;
- a Blue Cross/Blue Shield Plan utilizing subscriber premiums to partially settle a damage suit brought as a result of a paternity action against its CEO even though that CEO admitted paternity (p. 11).

Sopko noted that until the West Virginia failure, many regulators were mesmerized by voluntarism as a defensive ideology: "What is happening is that a lot of regulators have ignored the Blue Cross Plans because of the general assumption that Blue Cross is like motherhood, apple pie and the charitable hospital down the street, namely that there aren't any problems with it, there will never be any problems, it will always be there" (p. 19). The Subcommittee chair, Senator Sam Nunn, called this ideological halo "the non-profit syndrome" (p. 19).

The West Virginia debacle was resolved by the Blue Cross Plan in Cleveland taking over the failed Plan in West Virginia, plus another Blue Cross and Blue Shield Plan—one in good fiscal health—in that state. This was arranged in secret negotiations. The investigators were troubled by this secrecy. They noted that the Cleveland Plan's attorney cited an "old Sicilian saying that goes something like this: 'You get rich in the dark'" (U.S. Senate, 1992, July, p. 60). One thing discussed in the dark was, apparently, dumping some of the West Virginia subscribers, some steelworkers. In a phone conversation the Blue Cross attorney described how the Cleveland Plan could get out of honoring the steelworker contract that appeared to be unprofitable: "We have a insolvent plan. We will refuse to process claims, defend a breach of contract action and counter claim with a fraud complaint "(p. 60). This appears to set the profit needs of the Plan above the needs of subscribers.

These Subcommittee hearings led Donald Light, a medical sociologist and keen health care observer, to write a letter to the editor of The New York Times: "One comes away from the Nunn testimony with the impression that Blue Cross Plans are like Mafia families carving up the country into territories.... Moreover, by their own choice Blue Cross Plans no longer serve any significant public function. They are commercial companies in the guise of public interest, nonprofit institutions. Their self-perpetuating boards exhibit a striking lack of stewardship and public accountability" (Light, D., 1993, June 29, p. A14). This echoes Stuart's worst fears for the Blues in the 1950s: Blue Cross' identity merely cloaked self-seeking commercialism.

What had gone wrong? A failure of leadership to defend Blue Cross' institutional integrity. As Selznick cautions, "The leadership of any polity fails when it concentrates on sheer survival: institutional survival, properly understood, is a matter of maintaining values and distinctive identity" (1983, p. 63). When the Blues left "the community idea" behind in order to get ahead in the marketplace they jeopardized their distinctive identity. Profit-seeking had overwhelmed community service. And Tresnowski pointed out to his board that the Blues were drifting away from their mission and core values:

> We knew that certain qualities of leadership would define our future.... Leadership
> that was credible because it represented a set of values that had guided us for more
> than six decades. And out of that arose again the realizations that we had not come to
> grips with who and what we are.... We deferred on agreeing to a common mission,
> a deferral that has come back to haunt us.... By consciously avoiding our commit-
> ment to a common mission, we acted haltingly in Louisiana, New Jersey and Buffalo
> and indecisively in West Virginia.... In the long run it may not be important whether
> we are for-profit or not-for-profit. However, from the public's perspective, I don't
> think it's time to give up our non-profit status. Profits in health care and undue em-
> phasis on personal gains are large negatives in the context of health care reform.
> (Blue Cross and Blue Shield Association, 1992, pp. 3, 23)

Here Tresnowski was parting company with Rorem who had little faith in the profit motive to constructively guide providers or drive Blue Cross plans (Sigmond, 1985). In a 1992 nationwide advertising campaign, the Blues cloaked themselves in their nonprofit tradition and asserted that *they* (as opposed to their commercial competitors) were not motivated by economic gain.

Still, after fourteen years of business building, Tresnowski returned to institution building, "No individual or institution can be psychologically sound and maintain its integrity if it fails to define its identity and mission and to commit everyone of its energy to those purposes" (Blue Cross and Blue Shield Association, p. 24). Blue Cross leadership had been irresponsible. Responsible leadership can, Selznick observes, "be summarized under two headings: the avoidance of opportunism [i.e., unhealthy ideology] and the avoidance of utopianism" (1983, p. 143). These are the dangers of policy as ploy and plan. Opportunism is extreme ideology as ploy that disregards ethical principle or institutional identity. It is preoccupied with short-term gain and narrow self-centeredness. Instead of setting a clear mission, the organization is allowed to drift, reacting to various internal and external urges. It lives by exploitation. When leadership has no vision of a viable mission its character becomes dilute and disoriented. Selznick observes that such a character's "practical result is that the organization cannot perform any task effectively, and this weakens its ability to survive in the face of strong competition" (p. 145). Extreme utopianism, on the other hand, overgeneralizes purpose, Selznick gives an example: "Thus 'to make a profit' is widely accepted as a statement of purpose, but this is too general to permit responsible decision-making"

(p. 147). Utopian wishful thinking ignores the need for effective means to achieve purposes. Thus, mere exigency controls decision-making.

The Permanent Subcommittee on Investigations' inquiry reveals instances of irresponsible leadership. Its findings concerning Empire Blue Cross and Blue Shield of New York—then the nation's largest private health insurer with 7 million policy holders—illustrates unhealthy ideological leadership. Its findings concerning National Capital Blue Cross and Blue Shield (District of Columbia) illustrates unhealthy utopian leadership.

First, Empire Blue Cross. After six months of investigation the Subcommittee's staff found an incompetent and confused enterprise. They noted that Empire had "an inability to properly execute the most basic functions of an insurance company, resulting in abysmally poor service to subscribers and providers; a severe lack of internal controls, leading to a high degree of vulnerability to fraud; excessive expenditures for the benefit of senior officers and members of the board of directors; a propensity on the part of the plan management to blame external factors for the plan's failings and to rely upon external sources for relief to keep it afloat; inadequate oversight of management activities by the board of directors and ineffective regulation of the plan by the State Department of Insurance" (U.S. Senate, 1993, June 25, p. 5).

The staff also noted that the organization had failed to effectively define its mission and purpose, holding onto an out-of-date focus on hospital insurance as the marketplace rapidly grew to demand managed care and HMO products (1993, p. 166). The corporate culture under its just-resigned CEO was marked by his luxurious life-style and what one person described as a reign of terror (1993, p. 167). One example of the Plan's inability to adapt was its experience with HMOs. It started Healthnet, an HMO, in 1986. The HMO was ill-conceived and unappealing to consumers. Blue Cross raised its rates to cover the HMOs loses which only drove more HMO subscribers away, creating in turn more loses. By 1993 it accounted for only 3 percent of all HMO subscribers in the state (Meier, August 17, 1993).

Essentially, the Plan deceived New York State regulators into granting a rate hike to pay for the costs of Plan mismanagement. The Plan's executives had argued that commercial rivals were siphoning off the Plan's healthier individual policy holders. This "cherry picking" resulted in the Plan's community rate for individual (nongroup) subscribers to skyrocket.

Hence, they alleged, major loses. The Senate investigators found that the facts indicated otherwise. Essentially, the Plan "loss shifted," to coin a phrase, that is, they shifted losses suffered by the Plan in their poorly managed experience-rated group contracts and deceitfully called these community rate group loses. The Plan fudged the numbers. Hiding behind the Plan's traditional identity as a community service institution, the Plan's leaders gave the public doctored facts in order to maintain their own positions, pay, powers, and perks. This was policy as a deceitful defensive ideology—at the price of eroded legitimacy and identity. Belatedly, Empire's top management and board members were replaced. The Empire Blue Cross, although backward, was not truly conservative, because it had failed, in Dewey's terms to truly "absorb into its character" the idea of community service.

If the Subcommittee's report on Empire Blue Cross leaves one with an image not of empires but of obsolete big city political machines run by hacks delivering poor service while skimming off a bit of cream for themselves, its report on Blue Cross and Blue Shield of the National Capitol Area (District of Columbia) paints a picture of disastrous imperial adventures (Jan. 26–27, 1993). In 1986 the plan's CEO unveiled his vision of what he called "an empire" (p. 161). Basically, he careened down Mannix' swashbuckling path, but not anchored by Mannix' social values. This CEO, in Deweyan terms, "shut himself off from the established facts of life...[and turned] to the future before he [took] home to himself the meaning of the past" (1894). So began a futile, radical utopian adventure.

This irresponsible leader was unhappy, as were other Blue Cross CEOs, with how the loose Blue Cross and Shield confederation handled national accounts and related matters. His vision was to supplant the national association, hijack from the association the Blue Cross and Blue Shield trade marks and incorporate Blues subsidiaries around the globe. Plus, he would create the first regional Blue plan (merging his with those of Maryland, Virginia, and Delaware). This mid-Atlantic state behemoth, which he called "Big Mac," might then gobble up Blue plans in Arizona, Utah and West Virginia. The Board was hypnotized by this radical utopian master plan. This led to creating 45 (including 17 overseas) subsidiary corporations—where some subsidiaries created in turn further subsidiaries—which lost $100 million in a few years—much of these loses were in its HMO ventures. The leader's imperial vision soon led to the Plan becoming economically imperiled. When, this Blue Cross leader—now retired—was called to appear before the Senate Subcommittee, he pleaded the Fifth Amendment.

In terms of leadership, this failed grandiose adventure exemplifies the dangers of a radical utopian approach. This capricious vision was underpinned by an abstract idea that would, he assumed, melt away obstacles in his path. His successor recalls:

> It just seems to me that when the vision that he developed, which many of us initially, including me, thought was pretty dramatic, which he developed in the mid-eighties regarding diversification, I think that he became overwhelmed, or whatever it might be, with that concept, and it was a concept of growth. Growth, growth, growth was the view because he had a 20-year, as he called it, vision regarding where this company ought to be, needs to be.... For a long period, he really wasn't concerned about short-term results. He was concerned about the long-term view of this organization, and you can't be bothered with these issues. (p. 90)

Mesmerized by this magical and abstract concept of growth, the Plan created nearly four dozen for-profit subsidiaries without any real expertise or experience in these new lines. The CEO spent much of his time flying around the globe including twenty-two trips on the Concorde) wheeling and dealing. His salary tripled in a few years. The board was either ignorant or approved. There was no real accountability of management to the board, to the national association, or state regulators.

In 1988, board member Peter F. O'Malley—on leaving the board—saw, however, some of the underlying issues and tried to focus the board on the critical decision issue presented by the CEO's imperial vision: it was a choice between two corporate characters, that is, between its traditional not-for-profit care health insurance mission and this new for-profit enterprise. He pointed out that if the board chose the path of for-profit venturing, then that would require different skills of managing such a business, and a strategic plan—where the executives would need to be held accountable for achieving objectives. He was addressing the need to refine abstract ideals such as "growth" into achievable objectives, where there would be a practical plan to achieve those objectives. He called for responsible attention to *means*. The board disregarded his advice and allowed their Blue Cross and Blue Shield Plan to run amok—it drifted into utopian ruin without a strategic plan, nor appropriate managerial skills or structure. Years later, the CEO resigned and the board restructured with Mr. O'Malley as chair.

De-definition: Loss of Identity

Tresnowski in the 1990s pleaded with his trade association members for credible leadership, but plan misbehavior undermined that credibility. In 1993 *Time*, for example, reviewed instances of Blue Cross mismanagement and misconduct. Its article attempted an upbeat ending, citing various encouraging facts and figures issued by the Blues' association. But this was undermined by its last paragraph: "The problem is that such figures are furnished by the [Blue Cross] companies. Naturally if the numbers are fudged...then all tallies are suspect. And, as Senator Sam Nunn put it last week, 'If this nation is ever to truly reform its health-care system, we must find a way to hold insurers accountable to their subscribers, to regulators and to the public at large'" (R. Behar, July 12, 1993, p. 48). More recently, Tresnowski was grilled on CBS' "60 Minutes" program (May 15, 1994) where some Blue Cross and Blue Shield executives were depicted to the American public as incompetent and more interested in their own pay and perks than subscriber needs. Tresnowski attempted to defend his trade association board members but his facts and figures were refuted by the CBS reporter. The show cited a 1994 GAO report—based on current data provided by the Blue Cross and Blue Shield Association—that indicated that 25 percent of all Blue Cross and Blue Shield policyholders are subscribers with plans in poor financial condition (H. Rosenberg, May 15, 1994, pp. 7–8). This report raised basic questions about whether the national association as a trade association can effectively enforce its membership standards on the Blue Cross Plans. The role conflict is seemingly too severe. The association's board is made up of Blue Cross Plan CEOs. Its president works for the Plans he is charged to police. Indeed, some Blue Cross Plan CEOs believe that "the Association's trademark licensing functions should be performed by an independent body of non-Blues employees that would have the will to enforce the membership standards" (GAO, 1994, p. 17). This would be a move in the direction of Mannix' American Blue Cross with a national body chartered by the federal government in charge of protecting the social integrity of the Blue Cross brand and symbol. In February, 1995 Patrick Hays succeeded Tresnowski as Association president. Hays has a proven track record in managed care. He takes over a confederation that lost 10 million subscribers in the 1990s (Freudenheim, 1995) but also became the nation's leading HMO with a national enrollment (Kertesz, 1994) of 7.6 million HMO subscribers.

In 1994 the Blue Cross confederation was in the middle of its descent into de-definition. As Tresnowski noted: "If all health insurers play by the new rules, there will not be a unique role for the Blues. Many plans will merge or go out of business, but the strongest will survive and emerge even stronger" ("Blues are Merging," 1994). As the Blues get pulled into the commercial vortex, the confederation is being pulled apart. As one former Association official suggests: "There are internal contradictions in the system, and the [association] is not powerful enough to keep it all together. I would expect over time...we would end up with a handful of regional Blues" (Crenshaw & Priest, August 24–30, 1992).

In June of 1994 the Association's board made the critical decision of the Tresnowski era: it eliminated the nonprofit standard for membership. Now Blue Cross plans can convert to for-profit status, can compete with each other and the Association can promote for-profit enterprise (Blue Cross and Blue Shield Association, 1994). As a system the Blues are now characterless, lacking a common identity. They are simply sixty-eight business-oriented organizations joined together only by sharing the same trade mark. Tresnowski himself summarized the American health care blues on the last page of his last annual report: "But while we have a great opportunity to be the model [for American health care reform]...a major gap remains in our ability to define exactly who we are. As I complete my years as head of the Blue Cross and Blue Shield Association, I continue to regret that we have been unable to agree upon a common mission" (p. 16). Blue Cross had too much commercial sail with too little social mission anchor.

So the American health care *blues* is a lament about the loss of community mission and institutional identity amidst the endless *blue skies* of commercial opportunity—a dialectic between seeking self-hood and self-seeking. Still while Blue Cross is a symbol of these blues, it is more. For the *cross* is a symbol of community and service. Hence Blue Cross can still be a symbol of hopeful possibilities. This study is a hermeneutics which, like a looking glass, has critically reflected back on where Blue Cross has been. But "looking-glass" has another meaning besides that of a means of reflecting back one's image. it also is the name for just the clear glass section of a looking glass. So besides offering a look backwards, a hermeneutics also provides a look ahead, *through* the looking glass, to hopeful community-oriented possibilities.

5

Reconstruction: Turning to the Future

What is, then, a pragmatic view of the crisis in American health care policy? Let me begin with how we currently look at the situation. *USA Today* presents social science findings about public opinion concerning health care: "We love our doctors...and our hospitals...but dislike the system" (Anderson, K., 1991, March 11, p. 3B). As Kevin Anderson writes: "Nothing has shaped U.S. health care so much as our peculiarly American attitudes towards medicine, science, and government. Often these attitudes clash" (1991, March 11, p. 3B). Thus social science findings as communicated by the media leave us with the paradox that in general things are seen as a crisis, but in particular cases, things are fine. How can this be? What can we do about these "attitudes in conflict?" (Anderson, K., 1991, March 11, p. 3B).

Pragmatic theory suggests that there are four ways to deal with conflict: solve it, resolve it, absolve it, or dissolve it. Gharajedahi and Ackoff (1986) explain: "To *solve* a conflict is to select a course of action that is believed to yield the best possible outcome for one side at the cost of another.... To *resolve* a conflict is to select a course of action that yields an outcome that...minimally satisfies both of the opposing tendencies.... To *absolve* a conflict is to wait it out, to ignore it and hope it will go away.... Finally...to *dissolve* a conflict is to change the nature and/or environment of the entity in which it is embedded so as to create a win/win environment" (pp. 47–48).

Dissolving conflict is the Deweyan path. It is what he meant by "reconstructing" things. Reconstruction involves examining one's world view (ideological or utopian) and its assumptions, and this is done through a public process of participation. Only such a process can get rid of outworn world views that create conflict and hinder creative adjustment (Gharajedahi & Ackoff, 1986). Pragmatic learning, then, is a democratic participatory process of fact finding and sharing, reconceptionalizing problems and solutions. In a learning society, assumptions are always being challenged, organizations are "ideal-seeking" and citizens participate in a process to define these ideas (Gharajedahi & Ackoff, p. 53). This is society moved by "the democratic wish" (Morone, 1990).

So let us reconstruct the paradox of American public opinion on health care. For Dewey the problem of American politics is that industrialization and other social forces have created a "Great Society"—what we call "the system" (Dewey, 1976). The Great Society is our society as a vast system. The many are indoctrinated by the few, making a real public impossible. Dewey argues that a real public requires free "inquiry and publicity" (Dewey, 1976, p. 207)—not propaganda and secrecy.

When we tell pollsters that we give the U.S. health care system a poor grade, I suggest we are saying two things. First, we are repeating the media's message that our system is a mess—this is more propaganda than informed education—*and* we are saying that the system is part of a Great Society run by a cash nexus and we, vaguely feel troubled by this. There is something troubling in Ivan Boesky saying: "What good is the moon if you can't buy it or sell it?" (quoted in Blumberg, 1989, p. 207). Similarly, when we give good marks to *our* particular doctors and hospitals we are, I suggest, also saying two things. First, we are genuinely loyal to these face-to-face *community* providers (and this adds meaning to our lives). Second, we give them high grades because we are dependent on them for our health and sometimes for our lives. This reflects Dewey's satisfaction/satisfactory distinction. Many of us have our immediate medical needs met—we are satisfied. But we know that in the long run the present health care system is unsatisfactory. It lacks meaning and cannot be sustained. So the "public" opinion polls are not truly *public* in nature—because we are not yet a true public, but dependent elements of a Great Society. The "paradox" is merely a symptom of this problem: McNerney's North Star—community—has been eclipsed by Boesky's monetarized moon. Indeed, the polls actually deepen the problem by creating further alienation.

Gharajedahi and Ackoff (1986) point out that alienation is the biggest hurdle to a nation's developing productive, participatory processes. Alienation happens, they suggest, along five dimensions: powerlessness, incompetence, meaninglessness, exploitation, and values. Let me illustrate these points first in terms of opinion polls themselves and then a new health care problem: the mirage of insurance coverage.

The public opinion polls on health care attitudes put citizens into an atomized, fairly passive, powerless, responder role. The presentation of findings as a paradox increases a sense of ineffectualness as the problem-as-paradox appears unsolvable. People feel incompetent and defer to experts—yet the experts themselves only come up with unsolvable paradoxes rather than effective solutions. The situation as paradox puts meaning out of reach. The polls constantly reveal that the health system's benefits are unjustly distributed. People come to feel both exploited and left out—or fear being left out—for example, go uninsured. The polls and the press depict our values as in conflict. This raises doubt in the individual's mind as to his or her membership in a community.

The mirage of health insurance coverage is a new health care issue (Meirer, B., January 4, 1992). From 1988 to 1990, 400,000 seriously ill Americans found out that their health insurance policies were valueless. (Hence, millions of Americans statistically identified as covered by health insurance are effectively not, after all, protected.) These policies are sold by predatory schemes that are either incompetently or corruptly managed. These firms do not respond to policyholder claims, delay responding to claims or simply go out of business—leaving policyholders faced with tremendous bills.

In our industrialized society "people are conditioned to *get* things rather than *to do* them" (Illich, 1976, p. 214). When the impersonal health insurance system fails to provide promised benefits, the passive policyholder and others becomes profoundly alienated. The policyholder feels powerless and incompetent as he or she tries to correct for the health system failure. One person, the wife of a dying policyholder, describes her search for coverage: "It was like a nightmare. You didn't know where things began or ended" (Meirer, 1992, p. 28). When she turned to regulators she found out that they too are often powerless to keep these corrupt products out of the market, nor can they offer victimized customers an avenue of redress. One state regulator remarks: "There is nothing I can do and it makes me angry and frustrated" (Meirer, p. 25). The system appears meaningless to these people. A victim policyholder exclaims: "What happened to me is inconceivable to me. We're in the process of losing everything... what is going to happen down the road?" (Meirer, pp. 1, 23, 1992). One analyst describes the situation as a "netherland" (Meirer, p. 28) of fraudulent schemes and a "bewildering world" of regulatory loopholes and insurance industry obstacles.

People feel exploited by a health insurance industry confidence game and left adrift by the government.

Into this alienating picture of American health care a variety of "solutions" are noted in the media: managed care, HMOs, commercialized prepaid group practices, and so on. But in the media, and too often in policy, these "solutions" are not presented in the context of a richly and realistically nuanced social theory. The details of health policy issues are lost in the media's disenchanting coverage of health care political tactics.

Inquiry as Community Swarming

The way to dissolve the problem is to conduct proper inquiry. As Westbrook (1991) summarizes: "If the public was not to remain in eclipse, Dewey said, the Great Society had to be converted into what he termed the Great Community...and this was in the first instance a problem of inquiry and communication" (p. 309). "Inquiry and publicity" recalls McNerney's equation "Knowledge + Communication = Control." And it recalls his health care statesman who gets the facts and makes them public. To get a better understanding of inquiry and publicity, I want to go back to the starting point of our Blue Cross story— McNerney's Michigan study in the late 1950s—and give it an interpretation based on some of Marshall McLuhan's ideas (1972) that are very Deweyan.

First of all, in the late 1950s, Michigan's Governor G. Mennen Williams created a public commission to inquire into rising health care costs (this review relies on McNerney's 1984 AHA oral history volume). But the Commission needed facts to make intelligent decisions, so they asked McNerney at the University of Michigan to put together a study to come up with the facts. He then talked with a limited number of people in government, labor, management, health care, and members of the Commission before writing a grant proposal for a study to be submitted to the Kellogg Foundation. McNerney wrote the proposal quickly based on his experience as a health services administrator and researcher. McNerney recalls: "I think often how that creative process [of inquiry] is bastardized by involving too many people over too much time with too much money." My first point from McLuhan (1972, p. 236) is that McNerney, the swashbuckler, tried to organize his inquiries as *participatory raids*, bypassing standard bureaucratic operating procedures.

Second, McNerney, who was relatively inexperienced in research, pulled together a team (McNerney's emphasis) remarkable in its lack of credentialed expertise, but with members "with an intuitive feeling of the problem and with definitive questions born of experience" (McNerney, 1984) who got help when they required it. McLuhan's analogous points are illuminating here:

> Before a [World War II] commando raid was mounted, the practice was for officers and men to *confer as equals*.... Instead of approaching the problem from any particular point of view, they *swarmed* over the problem as a group, using their total knowledge as a group. [Preconceived] "blueprints" and "specifications" were scrapped.... The individual expert yielded to the wider range of perception provided by the corporate dialogue. (p. 236, italics added).

The point here is that social problems are solved here democratically. An "inclusive awareness" (McLuhan, 1972, p. 236) of a situation is gained by dialogical swarming—a community *grasps* the situation by a process of interacting with it and conferring about it.

Third is that McNerney, the swashbuckler, got the grant by going outside established procedures. He did not do an extensive literature review or involve a lot of people and pass things by various review committees. Here he avoids what McLuhan calls the "*Law of Implementation*: the newest awareness [prod] must be processed by the established procedures [pattern]." As McLuhan explains: "In the commando conference, those who were to implement the decisions were present and helped to make the discoveries that became the action" (p. 236).

Fourth was that the context of World War II created an environment that summoned commandos at the front and workers at home to see themselves as "actors in a drama" which converted work into participation, role-playing, and fun, the upshot of which, McLuhan suggests, was a level of productivity far exceeding that found in chain of command bureaucracies.

There is, however, one problem with the Michigan study as an example of inquiry: most of its provocative recommendations were not acted on. McNerney's study had fallen to the Law of Implementation after all. Like the Committee on the Costs of Medical Care, this commission was really only a *half-way* inquiry. It lacked effective communication, communication that would build support coalitions. This would have been obvious to either Franklin or Dewey. Inquiry lacked proper publicity. And in part this relates to the study not including *all* the appropriate "commandos." McLuhan points out: "In the commando conferences those who were to implement the decisions were present and helped to make the discoveries that became the action.... Its dialogue became dramatized. There was no question that once they had begun to confer they would fall back on the old command structure for implementation" (p. 236).

Conference recommendations will only be acted on in communities if it includes as participants people from all appropriate walks of life. McNerney's crew proves you do not need Ph.Ds. You do need people with burning questions and relevant experience and skills. More Michigan Commission recommendations would have been acted on if it included labor and business leaders, patients, other citizens, and people from the media—and if conferees have a sense of drama from knowing that *they* would *act* on the fruits of their dialogue.

Putting this in Deweyan terms, I want to suggest that the health care system's (i.e., the Great Society's) problems can only be addressed by communities that conduct "free inquiry...wedded to full and moving communication" (Dewey, 1976, p. 184). Moreover, since "community" with its needs and ideals is the key consideration for judging scientific findings, citizens rather than experts are the key participants. As Dewey wrote, sounding like Franklin's Poor Richard, "The man who wears the shoe knows best that it pinches and where it pinches" (1976, p. 207). Social scientists can help this process along. While Dewey wanted community inquiry to be sciencelike, he warned against, as Kaufman-Osborne (1985) and Westbrook (1991) emphasize, it being scientist led. Currently, a grassroots organizing effort is underway to convert local consumer discontent into pressure for health care reconstruction (Anderson, K., 1991, September 23).

As Kaufman-Osborne (1985) points out, social scientific verification was for Dewey social, indeed it was democratic. A finding was only true if a community could be persuaded to try it out and judge its utility. Thus a hypothesis must come out of social practice and be translated back into commonsensical language for it to be truly tested. As Kaufman-Osborne interprets Dewey, scientific "truth" is not verifiable by reference to methods or the agreement of fellow experts. Instead, for Dewey policy science must judge its findings in terms of ends-in-view "*worth* attaining under the given circumstances" (quoted in Kaufman-Osborne, p. 843, italics added).

Dewey argued that "finding out is not after all the same as knowledge.... The thing found out is truly known only when published, spread abroad, communicated, made effective in the common life, a bond of union among men" (quoted in Kaufman-Osborne, 1985, p. 842). Kaufman-Osborne suggests that Dewey saw social policy as enlightenment *and empowerment*. A central social scientific finding was for Dewey, as Kaufman-Osborne suggests, a reconstruction in commonsense language of a public's definition of a problematic situation. Such a redefinition opens the path to explore new possibilities of action. Such a redefinition expresses a problematically felt, but not yet grasped, problem—what Kaufman-Osborne calls a "disordered nexus of interrelated factors."

Let me compare the pragmatic vs. bureaucratic models with the list of opposites below.

Pragmatic	Bureaucratic/Great Society
prod	pattern
aggregate	segment
drama	routine
confer	order
participation	function
swarming	blueprint
action	behavior
improvisation	implementation
quick	slow
produce	process
community planners	expert planners
making known	finding out

Principled Adventure

The American health care system has gone from a too-small cottage "industry" at the start of this century to what will be a juggernaut enterprise approaching 20 percent of our GNP and jobs by the end of the century. Rosemary Stevens' (1989) question will then take on even larger ramifications. For whether health care becomes more like a school district or a public utility or a business may well, in turn, shape the overall structure and identity of America. Health care, for better or worse, is no longer a *fringe benefit*, but rather a *central society-defining institution*. So how we inquire and act about health care is more important than ever. My own hunch is that managed care and managed competition will not curb health care cost escalation. They are radical utopian ideas that put too much confidence in profits and managers and not enough in patients and providers. The access crisis will worsen.

In 1975 the Blue Cross Association published *A Guide to HMO Citizen Participation* (Miller) which made (unknowingly) a Deweyan case for HMOs conceptualized as more like school districts than as for-profit businesses. It stressed that HMOs were concrete, real places where consumers, managers, and providers interact. In Deweyan language, HMOs are face-to-face places in a community where neighbors can learn about and discuss common issues. The *Guide* suggested that HMOs could be intermediate organizations that would mediate between the individual and the health care system (the Great Society). It pointed to Group Health Cooperative in Seattle as an exemplary—if imperfect—democratic HMO. The *Guide* also criticized American acceptance of the technological imperative in health care and called for a change in our expectations of health care. It acted on Dr. Robert van Hoek's suggestion that what was needed is a citizen-driven, collective educational process. And it suggested that the HMO setting would be a good forum for this process. Recently, these themes have re-emerged.

I agree with Dr. Arnold Relman who, like Tresnowski, called for a fairer "simplified insurance system" (1990, p. 991). Like Tresnowski, he urged greater use of computers with respect to medical care. But Relman placed an emphasis not on policing current practices, but rather on assessing the efficiency of emerging technologies, procedures and practices. Also, Relman, unlike Tresnowski who is a managed care champion, endorsed prepaid group practice plans as his model for health care's future. He suggested that group practice is a sound way of organizing the delivery of care. It stresses, he argued, primary care, and these plans traditionally have had as their mission community service. Most strikingly in his proposal is his advocacy for "not-for-profit HMOs that are [governed] jointly by physicians and members" (p. 991). The *New York Times* (Egan, 1991, May 2, p. A12) similarly pointed to Seattle's consumer-owned Group Health Cooperative of Puget Sound as a model for democratic, accessible health care. It quoted Dr. Relman who argues: "with patients right on the board of directors monitoring them, doctors are committed to the highest quality of care. There's no incentive for doing more tests than indicated, but every incentive to do all that is indicated" (Egan, p. A12). The article focused on the half million member Group Health Cooperative as a "showpiece of health care democracy" which shows that "quality health care is not an impossible dream." Recently Kissick has argued that national reform around such prepaid group practices constitutes a "Benjamin Franklin Scenario" for health policy (1994).

We have gone from one demi-crisis to another for thirty years now. Hopping like "a mountain goat" (quoted in Anderson, 1968) from one nonsolution (Medicare/ Medicaid, HMO businesses, managed care) to another. Looking towards the twenty-first century, I want to suggest that we no longer need to fear Fishbein's "medical soviets" (communism does not work), but should look to build and join consumer governed prepaid group practices (democracy can work). This would be a uniquely American quest guided by a North Star of participatory democracy. We need to add a sentence to Walt Whitman's (Dewey's moral prophet) "By Ontario's Shore" that would attest to our quest to convert the Great Society's health care system into community. Whitman wrote:

> 0, I see flashing that this America is only you and me,
> Its power, weapons, testimony, are you and me.
> Its crimes, lies, thefts, defections, are you and me,
> Its congress is you and me, the officers, capitols,
> armies, ships are you and me.
> Its endless gestation of new states are you and me,
> The war (that was so bloody and grim, the war I will
> henceforth forget), was you and me,
> Freedom, language, poems, employments are you and me,
> Past, present, future, are you and me,
> I dare not shirk any part of myself,
> Nor any part of America good or bad...
>
> *The health care system is you and me.*
> *It is a shared adventure and responsibility.*

For Blue Cross and Blue Shield to be reconstructed, they need to rekindle their interest and investment in prepaid group practices. And they need a moral cause—policy as position—which mobilizes their communities to improve the quality of life. This is why I suggest that Blue Cross participate in the healthy cities movement in which people seek ways—policy as prod—to attain a level of health permitting them to lead socially satisfying and economically productive lives (J. Twiss, 1992, p. 105). Remember, Rorem would have preferred that Blue Cross been adopted by the nation's community chests and councils, not by the hospital industry. Blue Cross adopting the healthy community movement would help return the Blues to their community service destiny—policy as perspective. McNerney had privately envisioned a time when the Blues would diversify into quality of life areas such as transportation for the elderly, education for the chronically ill and housing for various groups (McNerney, 1984). This was his unfloated utopian idea. This quality of life consideration was the first new Blue Cross role concept since McNerney had introduced the control role concept in 1964. As Dewey said about responsible leadership: "The most progressive force in life is the idea of the past set free of its local and partial bonds and moving on to the fuller expression of its destiny" (1894). Community health—not commercial profits—should be the Blues' North Star.

References

Adams, J.A. (1986). *Voluntary associations* (J.R. Engel, ed.). Chicago: Exploration.

Alexander, T.M. (1987). *John Dewey's theory of art, experience and nature.* Albany, NY: State University of New York Press.

American Hospital Association (AHA) (1990). *Digest of national health care use and expense indicators.* Chicago: Author.

American Medical Association. (1959, January 17). Report of the Commission on Medical Care Plans. *Journal of the American Medical Association* (Special Edition).

American Medical Association. (1967a, June 18-22). *Proceedings of the House of Delegates—116 Annual Meeting.* Chicago: Author.

American Medical Association. (1967b, November 20). *Proceedings of the House of Delegates Meeting in Houston.* Chicago: Author.

AMA president-elect predicts big growth in group practice (1970, May 25). *AMA News,* p. 11.

Anderson, K. (1991, March 11). Why health care costs are tough to cure. *USA Today,* p. 3B.

Anderson, K. (1991, May 6). Health spending. *USA Today,* p. 3B.

Anderson, K. (1991, September 23). Health care administrative waste faces scrutiny. *USA Today,* p. 1B.

Anderson, O.W. (1968). *Health services in a land of plenty* (Health Administration Perspectives number A7). Chicago: Center for Health Administration Studies of the University of Chicago.

Anderson, O.W. (1975). *Blue Cross since 1929: Accountability and the public trust.* Cambridge, MA: Ballinger.

Anderson, O.W. (1985). *Health services in the United States: A growth enterprise since 1875.* Ann Arbor, MI: Health Administration Press.

Anderson, O.W. (1990). *Health services as a growth enterprise in the United States since 1875* (2nd Ed.). Ann Arbor, MI: Health Administration Press.

Auerbach, S. (1967, April 28). Group medicine said to lower costs. *Washington Post,* p. 1.

Backer, B. & van Steenwyk, J. (1969). *Draft prepaid group practice planning document.* New York: Martin E. Segal Co.

Backstage talk in the Capitol: Ground swell for prepaid group practice plans. (1967, May 15). *Washington Report on the Medical Sciences,* p. 1.

Barnard, C.I. (1938). *The functions of the executive.* Cambridge, MA: Harvard University Press.

Behar, R. (1993, July 12). Singing the Blue Cross Blues. *Time,* p. 48.

Bennis, W. (1989). *Why leaders can't lead: The unconscious conspiracy continues.* San Francisco: Jossey-Bass.

Benveniste, G. (1989). *Mastering the politics of planning: Crafting credible plans and policies that make a difference.* San Francisco: Jossey-Bass.

Blue Cross Association. (1964). *Annual report,* Chicago: Author.

133

Blue Cross Association. (1967a). *Annual report*. Chicago: Author.

The Blue Cross Association. (1967b, April 27). *Press release: Blue Cross president predicts spread of group practice, greater controls and planning to curb health cost rises.* Chicago: Author.

Blue Cross Association. (1967c, June 20). *Blue Cross Digest*. Chicago: Author.

Blue Cross Association. (1967d, June 23). *Minutes of Board Meeting*. Chicago: Author.

Blue Cross presses for study of prepaid groups. (1967e, August 4). *Medical World News*, pp. 28-29.

Blue Cross Association. (1967f, October 23). *Blue Cross Digest*. Chicago: Author.

Blue Cross Association. (1967g, October 25). *Blue Cross Digest*. Chicago: Author.

Blue Cross request for funds opposed. (1967h, December 11). *AMA News*, p. 5.

Blue Cross Association. (1970a). *Annual report*. Chicago: Author.

Blue Cross Association. (1970b, April 2). Proceedings of Workshop on Prepaid Group Practice in Bal Harbor. Chicago: Author.

Blue Cross Association. (1970c, April 3). *Minutes of Board of Governors special meeting on Blue Cross and group practice prepayment*. Chicago: Author.

Blue Cross Association. (1970d, June 9). *Proceedings of National Meeting on Alternative Forms of Health Care Delivery and Financing in Chicago*. Chicago: Author.

Blue Cross Association. (1970e, November 17-19). *Proceedings of National Meeting On Alternative Delivery Systems in Kansas City, MO*. Chicago: Author.

Blue Cross Association. (1971 a). *Annual report*. Chicago: Author.

Blue Cross Association. (1971b, August 12). *Minutes of The Board of Governors Meeting*. Chicago: Author.

Blue Cross Association, (1971c, November 2). *Transcript of testimony to Senate Subcommittee on Health*. Chicago: Author.

Blue Cross Association. (1972a). *ADS status report*. Chicago: Author.

Blue Cross Association. (1972b, May 10). *Transcript of testimony to the House of Representative's Committee on Interstate and Foreign Commerce—Subcommittee on Public Health and Environment*. Chicago: Author.

Blue Cross Association. (1973a). *Annual report*. Chicago: Author.

Blue Cross Association. (1973b, February 27). *Press release: New symbol heralds new era for nation's Blue Cross plans*. Chicago: Author.

Blue Cross Association. (1975). *Annual report*. Chicago: Author.

Blue Cross and Blue Shield Association. (1987). *Annual report*. Chicago: Author.

Blue Cross and Blue Shield Association. (1988). *Annual report*. Chicago: Author.

Blue Cross and Blue Shield Association. (1989). *Annual report*. Chicago: Author.

Blue Cross and Blue Shield Association. (1990). *Annual report*. Chicago: Author.

Blue Cross and Blue Shield Association. (1992). *Annual report to the plans*. Chicago: Author.

Blue Cross and Blue Shield Association. (1993, Oct. 15). A *pragmatic approach to health care Reform*. Chicago: Author.

Blue Cross and Blue Shield Association. (1993). *President's report*. Chicago: Author.

Blue Cross and Blue Shield Association (1993). *Delivering results in managed care*. Chicago: Author.

Blue Cross and Blue Shield Association (1994). *President's Report*. Chicago: Author.

Blues are merging and repositioning. (1994, April). *Hospital Strategy Report* 6(6): p. 8.

Blumberg, M. (1989). *The Predatory Society*. New York: Oxford Press.

Boorstin, D. (1987). *Hidden history*. New York: Harper & Row.

Boyte, H.C. (1991, Summer). Democratic engagement. *The American Prospect* (6), 55-66.

Breitwiser, M.R. (1984). *Cotton Mather and Benjamin Franklin*. New York: Cambridge University Press.

A bright prognosis for the once-frail HMOs. (1980, October 27). *Business Week*, pp. 111-116.

Brockway, R. (1990, June 11). Phone interview.

Brown, L.D. (1983). *Politics and health care organization: HMOs as federal policy*. Washington, D.C.: Brookings Institution.

Brown, L.D. (1987). (Ed.). *Health policy in transition*. Durham, NC: Duke University.

Brown, L.D. & McLaughlin, C. (1990, Winter). Constraining costs at the community level. *Health Affairs*, 9(4), 6-33.

Brown, L.D. (1991a). Capture and culture: Organizational identity in New York Blue Cross. *Journal of Health Policy, Politics and Law, 16*(4), 651-670.

Brown, L.D. (1991b). Review of *The democratic wish. Journal of Health Policies, Policy and Law, 16*(4), 817-21.

Buchanan, R. (1989). Declaration by design. In V. Margolin (ed.), *Design discourses* (pp. 91-109). Chicago: University of Chicago Press.

Burk, James. (1991). A pragmatic sociology. Introduction to M. Janowitz, *On social organization and social control* (pp. 1-56). Chicago: University of Chicago Press.

Burke, K. (1968). Dramatism. In D.L. Sills (ed.), *The international encyclopedia of the social sciences* (Vol. 7, pp. 445-52). New York: Macmillan.

Campbell, J. (1992). *The community reconstructs*. Carbondale, IL.: Southern Illinois University Press.

Campbell, J. (1995). *Understanding John Dewey*. Chicago: Open Court.

Cohodes, D.R. (1994, Spring). The slippery slope of health care reform. *Inquiry 31*(3): 4-9.

Committee On the Costs of Medical Care. (1932). *Final Report* (No. 28), adopted October 21 (Chicago: University of Chicago Press, 1933).

Crenshaw, A. & Priest, D. (1992, August 24-30). Insurer, health thyself. *The Washington Post Weekly Edition*, p. 20.

The crisis in health insurance. Part 1. (1990, August). *Consumer Reports*, pp. 533-549.

The crisis in health insurance. Part 2. (1990, September). *Consumer Reports*, pp. 608-617.

Deveney, K. (1988, February 15). What's ailing Blue Cross: Just about everything. *Business Week*, pp. 32-34.

Dewey, J. (1894). Reconstruction. In *John Dewey, The early works (Vol. 4)*: 90-105 (ed. Jo Ann Boydstron). Carbondale, IL: Southern Illinois University Press.

Dewey, J. (1925). *Experience and nature*. LaSalle, IL: Open Court.

Dewey J. (1955). Science and morals [excerpt from *Quest for certainty*]. In M. White (ed.) *The age of analysis* (pp. 178-188). New York: New American Library. (Orig. 1929.)

Dewey, J. (1958). *Art as experience*. New York: Capricorn. (Orig. 1934).

Dewey, J. (1963). *Liberalism and social action*. New York: Capricorn. (Orig. 1935).

Dewey, J. (1964). The nature of aims [excerpt from *Human nature and conduct*]. In R. Archambault (ed.) Dewey on education (pp. 70-107). New York: Random House. (Orig. 1922).

Dewey, J. (1976). *The public and its problems*. Chicago: Swallow Press. (Orig. 1927).

Dewey, J. (1991). *Lectures on ethics (1900-1901)* (ed. Donald F. Koch). Carbondale, IL: Southern Illinois University Press.

Digest of the Wilbur Committee's recommendations for changes in medical practice. (1932, November 30). *New York Times*, p. 10A.

Don't blame Blue Cross [Editorial]. (1991, August 12). *New York Times*, p. 14A.

Doherty, J. (1990, July 2). Phone interview.

Drucker, P.F. (1981). Behind Japan's success. *Harvard Business Review* (January-February) pp. 83-90.

Drucker, P.F. (1985). *Innovation and entrepreneurship*. New York: Harper & Row.

Drucker, P.F. (1987). The new meaning of corporate social responsibility. In McCarthy, D.J. (Ed.) *Business policy and strategy* (pp. 141-152). Homewood, IL: Irwin.

Duffus, R.L. (1932, December 4). Shall medicine be socialized? *New York Times*, Section 8, Part 2, p. 7.

Egan, T. (1991, May 2). Seattle showpiece of health care democracy. *New York Times*, p. A12.

Eilers, R.D. (1972, November 12). The impact of HMOs on Blue Cross and Blue Shield Plans. Delivered at the National Blue Cross and Blue Shield Actuarial Research Conference. Chicago.

Ellwood, P.J., Jr. (1970). *Presentation at the Blue Cross Association's National Meeting on Alternative Forms of Health Care and Finance*. Chicago, June 9.

Ellwood, P.M., Jr., Anderson, N.A. & Billings, J.E. Carlson, R., Hoagberg, E.J. & McClure, W. (1971, May-June). Health Maintenance Strategy. *Medical Care* (3), 291-298.

Elkin, S. (1987). Political institutions and political practice. In E.B. Portis, M.B. Levy, & M. Landau (Eds.) *Handbook of political theory and policy science* (pp. 111-125). Westport, CT: Greenwood.

Estes, C.L. (1994). Privitization, the welfare state and aging. In *The nation's health* (p. 138-148). (Eds. P.R. Lee & C. Estes & N. Ramsey). Boston: Jones and Bartlett.

Falkson, J.L. (1980). *HMOs and the politics of health system reform*. Chicago: American Hospital Association.

Falk, I.S. (1984). Interview by Lawrence Weeks. *Hospital Administration Oral History Collection*. Chicago: American Hospital Association.

Faltermayer, E.K. (1970, January). Better care at less cost without miracles. *Fortune*, pp. 80-83.

Feffer, A. (1987). *Between head and hand: Chicago pragmatism and social reform, 1886-1919*. Unpublished Ph.D. dissertation. University of Pennsylvania. Philadelphia, PA.

Feffer, A. (1993). *The Chicago pragmatists and American progressivism*. Ithaca, NY: Cornell University Press.

Feinstein, J. (1986). *A season on the brink: A year with Bobby Knight and the Indiana Hoosiers*. New York: Pocket Books.

Fialka, J. (1993, May 6). Washington battle for health reform showed possible erosion of Blue Cross/Blue Shield clout. *Wall Street Journal*, p. A 16.

Filene, E.A. (1929, October 19). Autocare vs. medical care. *Journal of the American Medical Association, 93*, 1247-49.

Fishbein, M. (1932, December 3). (Editorial) The Committee on the Costs of Medical Care. *Journal of the American Medical Association, 99*, 1950-52.

Fortune. (1970, January). Our ailing medical system. Author, pp. 79-99.

Foss, S.K., Foss, K.A. & Trapp, R. (1985). *Contemporary perspectives on rhetoric*. Prospect Heights, IL: Waveland.

Foster, M.S. (1989). *Henry J. Kaiser*. Austin: University of Texas.

Fox, D.M. (1986). *Health policies, health politics: The British and American Experience, 1911-1965*. Princeton, NJ: Princeton University Press.

Fox, D.M. (1993). *Power and illness*. Berkeley, CA: University of California Press.

Franklin, B. (1961). *The Autobiography and other writings* (ed. L.J. Lemish). New York: Signet.

Freudenheim, M. (1995, February 3). A new chief for National Blue Cross. The *New York Times*, p. C3.

Friedman, E. (1982, December 16). Profile: Guiding Blue Cross and Blue Shield through troubled waters, *Hospitals*, pp. 91-96.

Friedmann, J. (1987). *Planning in the public domain: From knowledge to action.* Princeton, NJ: Princeton University.

Fuller, L.L. (1981). *The principles of social order.* [Ed., Kenneth I. Winston]. Durham, NC: Duke University Press.

Gardner, J.W. (1963). *Self-renewal: The individual and the innovative society.* New York: Norton.

Gardner, J.W. (1965, October). How to prevent organizational dry rot. *Harper's*, pp. 20-26.

Gardner calls group practice conference. (1967, October 2). *AMA News.*

Garland, S. (July 20, 1992). A black eye for the blues? *Business Week*, p. 33.

GAO. (1994, April). *Blue Cross and Blue Shield: Experiences of weak plans underscore the role of effective state oversight.* Washington, D.C.: U.S. General Accounting Office.

Gharajedaghi, J. & Ackoff, R.L. (1986). *A prologue to national development planning.* Westport, CT: Greenwood Press.

Ginzberg, E. (1990). *The medical triangle.* Cambridge, MA: Harvard.

Gossett, J.W. (1972, September 11). Look who's pushing prepaid practice now. *Medical Economics*, pp. 171-189,

Gove, P.H. (ed.). (1986). *Webster's new international dictionary.* (3rd Edition). Springfield, MA: Merriam-Webster.

Hale, J.A. & Hunter, M.M. (1988, June). *From HMO movement to managed care industry: The future of HMOs in a volatile health care market.* Excelsior, MN: InterStudy.

Halberstam, D. (1986). *The reckoning.* New York: Morrow.

HCSC introduces national HMO network. (1982, March). *Basically Business.* Chicago: Health Care Service Corporation. p. 1.

A health insurer that needs a cure. (1982, May 10). *Business Week*, pp. 158, 163-64.

Health Policy Advisory Center. (1971). *The American health empire: Power, profits, and Politics.* New York: Vintage.

Hedinger, F.R. (1968). The social role of Blue Cross. *Inquiry 5*(2), 3-12.

Henry, M.E. (1974, October). *Alternative delivery systems prospectus.* Chicago: Blue Cross Association.

Here's a president who criticizes his own outfit. (1971, February). *Forbes*, p. 48.

Hickman, L.A. (1990). *John Dewey's pragmatic technology.* Bloomington: University of Indiana.

Hollander, N. (1990, June 7). Phone interview.

Illich, I. (1976). *Medical nemesis.* New York: Pantheon.

Iglehart, J.K. (1982, August 12). Health policy report: The future of HMOs. *New England Journal of Medicine, 307,* 451-456.

Insider interview: B.R. Tresnowski (1989, December 4). *Health Week*, pp. 10-13.

The Investor's guide to HMOs. (DHHS publication No. PHS 83-50202). Washington, D.C.: U.S. Government Printing Office.

Jacobson, S. (1991, May 6). Doctors, patients trade blame. *USA Today*, p. 1.

Janowitz, M. (1978). *The last half-century: Societal change and politics in America.* Chicago: University of Chicago Press.

Kaufman-Osborne, T.V. (1985). Pragmatism, policy science, and the state. *American Journal of Political Science, 29* (November), 826-849.

Kearney, R. (1991). Between tradition and utopia. In *On Paul Ricoeur*, p. 74–83 (ed. David Wood). New York: Routledge.

Kertesz, L. (1994, Sept. 12). A Blue streak for managed care. *Modern Hospital*.

Ketchum, R. (1966). *Benjamin Franklin*. NY, NY: Washington Square Press.

Kirshner, E. (1989, November 6). Blues try to pull it all together. *Health Week*, pp. 8–9.

Kissick, M.L. (1994). *Medicine's dilemmas*. New Haven, CT: Yale.

Klein, E.A. (1966). (Ed.). *A complete etymological dictionary of the English language*. New York: Elsevier.

Kloppenberg, J.L. (1986). *Uncertain victory: Social democracy and progressivism in European and American thought*. New York: Oxford.

Koch, H. & Miller, S.I. (1940). *The Sea Hawk*. Hollywood, CA: Warner Brothers.

Law, S.A. (1974). *Blue Cross: What went wrong?* New Haven, CT: Yale University Press.

Levine, R.A. (1968). Rethinking our social strategies. *The Public Interest, 10* (Winter), 86–96.

Levine, R.A. (1972). *Public planning: Failure and redirection*. New York: Basic Books.

Lewin, T. (1991, April 28). High medical costs hurt growing numbers in U.S. *New York Times*, pp. 1A & 14A.

Light, D.W. (1991). The restructuring of the American health care system. In T.J. Litman & L.S. Robins (Eds.) *Health Politics and Policy* (pp. 53–65). Albany, NY: Delmar.

Light, D.W. (1993, June 29). Blue Cross turns into a national scandal. *New York Times*, p. A14.

Litman, T.J. & Robins, L.S. (1991). *Health Politics and Policy*. Albany, NY: Delmar.

Locin, M. (1991, March 7). Russo bill calls for universal health insurance. *Chicago Tribune*, p. 3.3.

Lofland, J & Lofland, L. (1984). *Analyzing social settings*. (2nd ed.). Belmont, CA: Wadsworth.

Lundberg, G.L. (1991, May 15). National health care reform: An aura of inevitability is upon us. *The Journal of the American Medical Association, 265*, 2566–2567.

Lyles, M.A. & Thomas, H. (1988). Strategic problem formulation. *Journal of Management Studies, 25*(3), 131–146.

MacColl, W.A. (1966). *Group practice and prepayment of medical care*. Washington, D.C.: Public Affairs.

Macek, C.F. (1983). Review of *The Sea Hawk*. In *Magill's American Film Guide*, Vol. 4 (ed., F.N. Magill) pp. 2892–2893. Englewood, NJ: Salem.

Majchrzak, A. (1984). *Methods for policy research*. Beverly Hills, CA: Sage.

Majone, G. (1989). *Evidence, arguments and persuasion in the policy process*. New Haven, CT: Yale.

Majority of business coalitions engaged in HMO-related activities. (1982, October). *Group Health News, 23*(10), p. 1.

Majority would change health coverage to control costs *New York Times* finds. (1982, May). *Group Health News, 23*(5), p. 9.

Mannix, J. (1944). Why not an American Blue Cross? *Hospitals*, April.

Mannix, J. (1959, November 1). Prepayment, Hospitals and the Future. *Hospitals, 33*, pp. 40–44 & 123.

March, J.G. & Olsen, J.P. (1989). *Rediscovering institutions: The organizational basis of politics*. New York: The Free Press.

Marmor, R.T. & Schlesinger, M. & Smithey, R.W. (1994). Nonprofit organizations and health care. In *Understanding health care reform* (pp. 48–85), T.R. Marmor. New Haven, CT: Yale.

Marsh, V. (1990, July 30). Phone interview.

Mayer, M. (1949, November). The rise and fall of Dr. Fishbein. *Harper's*, pp. 76-85.

McCarthy, D.J., Minichiello, R.J. & Curran, J.R. (1987) (eds.). *Business policy and strategy*. Homewood, IL: Irwin.

McLuhan, M. & Newitt, B. (1972). *Take today: The executive as drop out*. New York: Harcourt, Brace, Javanovich.

McKeon, R. (1987). *Rhetoric: Essays in invention and discovery*. M. Bachman (ed.). Woodbridge, CT: Ox Bow.

McNary, W.S. (1959, November 1). How Blue Cross can explain hospital costs. *Hospitals, 33*, pp. 46-50 & 123.

McNerney, W.J. (1964). The role of Blue Cross in cost and quality controls. In *Can voluntary controls do the job: Proceedings of the 7th Annual Symposium on Hospital Affairs*. (pp. 49-55). Chicago: University of Chicago Graduate School of Business.

McNerney, W.J. (1965, October 21). The future of voluntary prepayment for health services. *New England Journal of Medicine, 273*, 907-914.

McNerney, W.J. (1966). *Comprehensive personal health services: A management challenges the health professions*. Remarks presented at the 94th Annual Meeting of the American Public Health Association, October 31, San Francisco.

McNerney, W.J. (1967a, August 23). Transcript of remarks on receiving the Justin Ford Kimball Award from the American Hospital Association. Chicago.

McNerney, W.J. (1967b). Interview. *In Hospitals, 41* (July 1), pp. 49-54.

McNerney, W.J. (1969, June 5). The health administration establishment: Underachiever. Speech given at the 19th Annual Group Health Institute. New York.

McNerney, W.J. (1970, April 1-2). *Blue Cross and group prepayment: Policy paper delivered at Annual Meeting of the Plans*. Chicago: Blue Cross Association.

McNerney, W.J. (1977). Two sides of the same coin: Voluntary financing and voluntary management. *Hospital and Health Services Administration*, Summer, 58-74.

McNerney, W.J. (1979). *The private sector perspective on health planning*. Presented at American Health Planning Association Annual Meeting. San Francisco.

McNerney, W.J. (1982). *Comment*. In R.C. Rorem, *A quest for certainty*. (pp. xi-xiii). Ann Arbor, MI: Health Administration Press.

McNerney, W.J. (1983). The evolution in health services management. In D. Mechanic (ed.) *Handbook of health, health care, and the health professions* (pp. 523-535). New York: The Free Press/Macmillan.

McNerney, W.J. (1984). Interview by Lawrence Weeks. *Hospital Administration Oral History Collection*. Chicago: American Hospital Association.

McNerney, W.J. (1990, May 17). Interview.

Meier, B. (1992, January 4). A growing U.S. Affliction: Worthless health policies—insurance mirage. *New York Times*, pp. 1 and 28A.

Meier, B. (1993, August 17). Blue Cross tries to push plans for managed care. The *New York Times*, p. A12.

Meyer, E.M. (1977, April). Renewed voluntary spirit needed says Blue Cross. *Modern Healthcare*, pp. 56-57.

Meyers, H.B. (1970, January). The medical-industrial complex. *Fortune*, pp. 90-91.

Miles, M.B. & Huberman, A.M. (1984). *Qualitative data analysis*. Beverly Hills, CA: Sage.

Millenson, M.L. (1991, July 10). Time of reckoning in care crisis. *Chicago Tribune*, p. 1.

Millenson, M.L. (1991, September 6). Healthcare revamp predicted. *Chicago Tribune*, p. 3.1.

Millenson, M. (1993, August 10). Blue Cross fights fever of scandal. *Chicago Tribune*, pp. 1 & 8.

Miller, I. (1974). *A guide to HMO cooperative planning.* Chicago: Blue Cross Association.

Miller, I. (1975). *HMO consumer participation... why, how, and where it leads.* Chicago: Blue Cross Association.

Miller, I. (1990). Health policy analysis as ideology and as utopian rhetoric: The case of U.S. Federal Health Maintenance Organization policy analysis. *Business and Professional Ethics Journal, 9*(3 & 4), 173–182.

Miller, I. (1993). A pragmatic health policy tradition. *Business and Professional Ethics Journal, 12*(1): 47–57.

Mintzberg. H. (1987, Fall). The strategy concept I: Five Ps for strategy. *California Management Review, 30*(1), 11–28.

Morone, J. (1990). *The democratic wish.* New York: Basic Books.

National Association of Blue Shield Plans. (1967a, June 18). *Minutes of Executive Committee Meeting.* Chicago: Author.

National Association of Blue Shield Plans. (1967b, July 25). *Minutes of Executive Committee Meeting.* Chicago: Author.

Navarro, V. (1990). Medical history as justification rather than explanation. In J.W. Salmon (ed.) *The corporate transformation of health care* (pp. 213–232). Amityville, NY: Baywood.

Nisbet, R. (1988). *The present age: Progress and anarchy in modern America.* New York: Harper & Row.

Non-profit HMOs retain tax exempt status. (1986, September-October). *Group Health Association of America News, 27*(9 & 10), 10.

Ortoney, A. (1979). (Ed.). *Metaphor and thought.* New York: Cambridge.

Padgug, R.A. (1991). Afterword: Empire Blue Cross and Blue Shield as an object of historical analysis. *Journal of Health Politics, Policy and Law, 16*(4), 793–816.

Perlmutter, H.V. (1965). *Towards a theory and practice of social architecture: Building indispensable institutions.* London: Tavistock.

Pettigrew, A. (1983). On studying organizational cultures. In J. Van Maanen (ed.). *Qualitative methodology* (pp. 87–104). Beverly Hills, CA: Sage.

Pettigrew, A. (1987). Context and action in the transformation of the firm. *Journal of Management Studies, 24*(6), 649–676 (November).

Pettigrew, A., McKee, L., & Ferlie, E. (1988). Understanding change in the NHS. *Public Administration, 66*(3), 295–317.

Phillips, K. (1990). *The politics of rich and poor.* New York: Random House.

Phillips, S. (1989, May 22). Humana regains that healthy glow. *Business Week,* pp. 127–28.

PHS rejects BCA request for PGP study funds. (1968, May 6). *AMA News,* p. 8.

Pulliam, S. (1991, March 3). Blue Cross collapse in West Virginia puts many in dire straits. The *Wall Street Journal,* p. 1.

Relman, A.S. (1980). The new medical-industrial complex. *New England Journal of Medicine, 303,* 963–970. (October 23, 1980).

Relman, A.S. (1990). Reforming the health care system. *New England Journal of Medicine, 323,* 991–992. (October 4).

Richman, L.S. (1983, May 2). Health benefits come under the knife. *Fortune,* pp. 95–110.

Ricoeur, P. (1986). *Lectures on ideology and utopia.* (G.H. Taylor, ed.). New York: Columbia.

Ricoeur, P. (1991). *From text to action.* (K. Blamey & J.B. Thompson, Eds.) Evanston, IL: Northwestern Illinois Press.

Riedell, D.C., Walden, D.C. & Meyer, S.M. (Eds.). (1984). *Use of health care resources.* Ann Arbor: Health Administration Press.

Robert Wood Johnson Foundation (1995). *Investigation awards in health policy.* Princeton, NJ.

Rogin, M. (1959). *Voluntarism as an organizational ideology.* Unpublished MA Thesis, Chicago: University of Chicago.

Rogin, M. (1962). Voluntarism: The political functions of an anti-political doctrine. *Industrial and Labor Relations Review, 15* (July), 521-35.

Rorem, R.C. (1982). *A quest for certainty.* Ann Arbor, MI: Health Administration Press.

Rorem, R.C. (1988, November 5). Insurance, competition, and physician fees. *Hospitals*, p. 120.

Rorty, R. (1989). *Contingency, irony, and solidarity.* New York: Cambridge.

Rosenberg, C.L. (1971, November 8). The Blues are rolling out their own HMO bandwagon. *Medical Economics*, p. 267.

Rosenberg, H. (1994, May 15). *60 Minutes*: Blue Cross Blue Shield. XXVI(35): 2-8. NY: CBS News.

Ross, D. (1991). *The origins of American social science.* New York: Cambridge.

Salmon, J.W. (1975). The health maintenance organization strategy: A corporate takeover of health care delivery. *International Journal of Health Services, 5*, 609-624.

Salmon, J.W. (1990). (ed.). *The corporate transformation of health care: Issues and directions.* Amityville, NY: Baywood Publishing Company.

Sanders, M.K. (Ed.). (1960, October). The crisis in American medicine [special supplement]. *Harper's*, pp. 123-174.

Schein, E.H. (1969). *Process consultation: Its role in organization development.* Reading, MA: Addison-Wesley.

Schon, D. (1971). *Beyond the stable state.* New York: Norton.

Schon, D. (1979). Generative metaphor: A perspective on problem-setting in social policy. In A. Ortony (Ed.), *Metaphor and thought* (pp. 254-283). New York: Cambridge University.

Schorr, D, (1970). *Don't get sick in America.* Nashville: Aurora.

Schultze, C.L. (1977). *The public use of private interest.* Washington, D.C.: Brookings Institution.

Selznick, P. (1983). *Leadership in administration* (paperback edition with new preface). Berkeley, CA: University of California Press (1957).

Selznick, P. (1992). *The Moral Commonwealth.* Berkeley, CA: University of California Press.

Sheffield, R. (1969, September). The Harvard experiment. *Perspective*, pp. 7-13.

Sibery, E. (1988). Interview by Lawrence Weeks. *Hospital Administration Oral History Collection.* Chicago: American Hospital Association.

Sibery, E. (1990, August 6). Phone interview.

Sigmond, R.C. (1982). *Comment.* In R.C. Rorem, *A Quest for Certainty* (pp. 59-61). Ann Arbor: MI.

Sigmond, R. (1990, May 10). Interview.

The spiraling costs of health care. (1982, February 8). *Business Week*, pp. 58-61.

Starr, P. (1982). *The social transformation of American medicine.* New York: Basic Books.

Starr, P. (1990, July 23). Good offices [Review of *Bureaucracy*, J. Wilson, Basic, 1989] *New Republic*, pp. 39-41.

Stevens, R. (1971). *American medicine and the public interest.* New Haven: Yale.

Stevens, R. (1989). *In sickness and in wealth: American hospitals in the twentieth century.* New York: Basic Books.

Stevens, R. (1991a). The hospital as a social institution. *Hospitals and Health Services Administration, 36*, 163-173.

Stevens, R. (1991b). Can the government govern? *Journal of Health Politics, Policy, and Law, 16*(2), 281–306.

Stewart, C. & Smith, C. & Denton, R.E. (1984). *Persuasion and social movements.* Prospect Heights, IL: Waveland.

Stewart, D. (1987). Interview by Lawrence Weeks. *Hospital Administration Oral History Collection.* Chicago: American Hospital Association.

Stewart, D. (1990, June 21). Phone interview.

Stone, D. (1988). *Policy paradox and political reason.* Glenview, IL: Scott, Foreman and Company).

Strumpf, G. (1990, June 22). Phone interview.

Stuart J. (1953, August). Blue Cross slips are showing. *The Modern Hospital, 81*(2), 52–54.

Stuart, J. (1959, February 16). Blue Cross and insurance. *Hospitals, 33,* 51–54.

The time is ripe for community initiatives and new ideas. (1982). *Group Health News, 23*(3), 10.

Tresnowski, B.R. (1985, Spring). Conventional and alternative health care delivery systems. *Health Matrix, 3*(1), 3–5.

Tresnowski, B.R. (1986). Interview by Lawrence Weeks. *Hospital Administration Oral History Collection.* Chicago: American Hospital Association.

Twiss, J.M. (1992, Spring-Summer). California healthy cities project. *National Civic Review, 81*(2): 105–114.

United States Senate Subcommittee on Investigations. (1992, June 25 & 30). *Hearings: Oversight of the insurance industry—Blue Cross/Blue Shield Empire Plan (New York).* Washington, D.C.: Government Printing Office.

United States Senate Subcommittee on Investigations. (1992, July 2, 29 & 30). *Hearings: Efforts to combat fraud and abuse in the insurance industry* (Washington, D.C.: Government Printing Office.

United States Senate Subcommittee on Investigations. (1992, September 24-25). *Hearings: Oversight of the insurance industry—Blue Cross/Blue Shield Maryland Plan.* Washington, D.C.: Government Printing Office.

United States Senate Subcommittee on Investigations. (1992, 1993, January 26-27). *Hearings: Oversight of the insurance industry—Blue Cross/Blue Shield National Capital Area.* Washington, D.C.: Government Printing Office.

United States General Accounting Office. (1994, April). *Blue Cross and Blue Shield: Experiences of weak plans underscores the role of effective state oversight.* Washington, D.C.: Government Printing Office.

VanSteenwyk, J. (1975a, May 5). HMOs: A bandwagon. *ADS Bulletin.* Chicago: Blue Cross Association.

VanSteenwyk, J. (1975b, September 17). *HMOs and national accounts: Remarks at BCA national HMO system work group meeting.* Chicago.

VanSteenwyk, J. (1975c, October 23). High road or load road. *ADS Bulletin.* Chicago, Blue Cross Association.

Veney, J. (1990, June 7). Phone interview.

Vincent, G. (1896, January). The province of sociology. *American Journal of Sociology, 1,* 488.

Vladeck, B.C. (1985, Summer). The dilemma between competition and community service. *Inquiry, 22,* 115–121.

Walker, F. (1979). American versus sovietism. *Bulletin of the History of Medicine, 53,* 488–504.

Wasik, J.F. (1991, July/August). The crisis in health insurance. *Consumer Digest*, pp. 49–64.

Weber, M. (1958). *The Protestant ethic and the spirit of capitalism*. T. Parson (trans.). New York: Scribners (Orig. 1904–1905).

Weber, M. (1964). *The sociology of religion*. E. Fischoff. Trans. Boston: Beacon Press (Orig. 1922).

Westbrook, R.B. (1991). *John Dewey and American democracy*. Ithaca, NY: Cornell University.

Western, J. (1967, August 28). What's behind credit card medicine? *The National Observer*, p. 1.

Whiteis, D. & Salmon, W.J. (1987). The proprietarization of health care and the underdevelopment of the public sector. *International Journal of Health Services, 17*, 47–56.

Wiebe, R. (1975). *The segmented society: An introduction to the meaning of America*. New York: Oxford.

Will, G.F. (1990). *Suddenly: The American idea abroad and at home*. New York: The Free Press/Macmillan.

Williams, W.H. (1976). *America's first hospital: The Pennsylvania Hospital 1751–1841*. Wayne, PA: Haverford House Publishers.

Wilson, J. (1989). *Bureaucracy*. New York: Basic Books.

Wright, E. (1986). *Franklin of Philadelphia*. Cambridge, MA: Belknap-Harvard.

Yin, R. (1984). *Case study research*. Beverly Hills, CA: Sage.

Index